The Rhythm Is Life

OrangeBooks Publication

1st Floor, Rajhans Arcade, Mall Road, Kohka, Bhilai, Chhattisgarh 490020
Website: **www.orangebooks.in**

First Edition, 2025

ISBN: 978-93-6554-450-3

Price: Rs. 399.00

Printed in India

THE RHYTHM IS LIFE

A FITNESS JOURNEY THAT STARTS FROM WITHIN AND MOVES IN RHYTHM.

KUNDAN AJAY SHARMA

OrangeBooks Publication
www.orangebooks.in

Contents

Introduction

Dear reader,

Before we truly begin, I invite you gently to pause. If it feels comfortable, close your eyes. Let one breath arrive and then leave, without needing to change it. Notice the rise and fall of your chest as your diaphragm descends on the inhale and eases back on the exhale. You might sense your ribs widening slightly, your abdomen softening, and if you listen closely the subtle variability in your heartbeat. That natural ebb and flow, sometimes called respiratory sinus arrhythmia, is one way the heart and lungs coordinate moment by moment. Ask your shoulders whether they'd like to lower a little. Ask your jaw if it's ready to release what it has been holding. And ask your mind, often racing ahead or replaying what has passed, if it might arrive here, now, in this single breath, with no requirement to be anywhere else. In this unhurried pause, free of urgency, pressure, or judgment, allow yourself to come home to yourself, just as you are.

Perhaps you picked up this book because you've tried many times before. You may have measured meals, tracked steps, experimented with programs that promised transformation, and followed detailed rules about what to eat, how intensely to move, and exactly when to rest. For a time, those efforts might have produced visible changes: pounds lost, strength gained, numbers moving in the direction you hoped. And yet, beneath the discipline and the metrics, a fragile tension can remain, the worry that if you loosen your grip, miss a day, or exhale a bit too long, the progress might slip away. It is exhausting to live as if your body were an adversary to be controlled or conquered.

This is deeply understandable. We live in a culture that often equates self-worth with output and celebrates conquest of markets, milestones, even our own biology. We're taught to treat hunger as a flaw to suppress, stillness as laziness to correct, and discipline as valid only when it feels punishing. In the process, we can confuse force with strength and begin to see the body as something separate: stubborn, defective, endlessly in need of fixing. When the body finally resists fatigue, pain, illness, or quiet signals we struggle to name, we may blame ourselves for "lacking willpower" rather than pausing to ask what these signals have been trying to communicate all along.

But what if health is not something to wrestle into place? What if your body already contains robust, built-in capacities for repair and adaptation, and what it most needs is not more control, but more connection, more kindness, more consistent space to respond to life's demands? Research across physiology and psychology suggests that sustainable change tends to emerge when practices are repeated with clarity and compassion, when stress and recovery are balanced, and when motivation is supported by meaning rather than fear. In other words, many people find that lasting fitness is less about iron willpower and more about rhythm.. trustworthy, gentle repetition that gradually becomes part of who you are.

This book invites you into a different way. Not softer because you are fragile, but wiser because you are human. Your body is not a machine to hack, punish, or "optimize" into submission. It is a living, breathing network of twelve interrelated systems like respiratory, nervous, circulatory, muscular, skeletal, digestive, endocrine, immune, urinary, lymphatic, integumentary, and reproductive, each designed to support the others in an ongoing conversation. Health is not produced by forcing one part to work harder in isolation; it unfolds when these systems can coordinate smoothly, adapting to your daily life through processes often described as homeostasis (maintaining internal stability) and allostasis (achieving stability through change). When one system is supported, its benefits can ripple across the others: steadier breathing can influence the nervous system, which in turn shapes heart rhythm, muscular recovery, digestion, immune readiness, and sleep quality. None of this guarantees any single outcome, and it never replaces individualized medical care but understanding these relationships can help you work with your body rather than against it.

Throughout these pages, you will be offered simple, human practices rooted in how the body functions. Breathing with awareness can help regulate carbon dioxide and oxygen balance, guide the diaphragm's movement, and signal safety to the autonomic nervous system. Gentle, regular movement builds strength and mobility while supporting circulation and joint health; it also affects mood and motivation through well-studied neurochemical pathways. Consistent, unhurried sleep supports metabolic regulation, memory, tissue repair, and immune function. Nourishing food that is chosen with gratitude rather than fear provides the raw materials for hormones, enzymes, neurotransmitters, and cellular repair. None of these practices need to be extreme to be effective; their power comes from rhythm and repeatability. Complex rules are not prerequisites for change. What helps most people over time is pacing that you can live with, practices you can enjoy, and small decisions that are easy to return to when life gets busy.

You may also recognize why consistency can be so challenging. Discipline that relies on pressure alone is difficult to sustain because it keeps the body and mind in a defensive stance. The nervous system tends to adhere more readily to routines that feel safe and meaningful. Pleasure and confidence are not indulgences; they are practical tools for learning. Habits are more likely to stick when the cues are clear, the effort is manageable, and the rewards feel immediate enough to notice an ease in your breath, steadier energy, a sense of agency. Over time, repetition wires patterns of attention and action, and those patterns become increasingly automatic. In this way, rhythm is not merely poetic language; it is a physiologic and psychological ally.

We will begin just as life begins, with the breath. Breathing is both automatic and trainable, a bridge between body and mind. On inhalation, the diaphragm contracts and moves downward, allowing the lungs to expand as air travels through the nose or mouth, down the trachea, and into branching bronchi and bronchioles that end in alveoli, the tiny air sacs where gas exchange occurs. On exhalation, the diaphragm relaxes and rises. Breathing through the nose, when possible, can warm and humidify air, filter particles, and introduce small amounts of nitric oxide generated in the nasal passages; this gas can help dilate airways and blood vessels locally, supporting efficient airflow and oxygen delivery. Slow, comfortable breathing patterns especially when the exhale is unforced and slightly longer than the inhale it can help nudge the autonomic nervous system toward a calmer state for many people, sometimes reflected in increased heart-rate variability, a marker associated with adaptability. These effects are not universal and are not a cure for medical conditions, but they illustrate how deliberate breath can influence multiple systems at once.

From the breath, we will move system by system not to micromanage the body, but to listen more closely to what each part needs and how it collaborates with the rest. The nervous system helps you detect and respond to stressors and safeties alike; the circulatory system delivers oxygen and nutrients while carrying away by-products; the muscular and skeletal systems provide structure and movement; the digestive system absorbs and processes fuel; the endocrine system coordinates longer-range signals through hormones; the immune system identifies and addresses threats while learning from past exposures; the urinary and lymphatic systems support fluid balance and waste clearance; the integumentary system that is the skin, hair, and nails that protects and senses; and the reproductive system sustains generational continuity and influences health across the lifespan. Each of these systems adapts daily through feedback loops. When we support them in a thoughtful sequence, starting with foundations like breath, sleep, and gentle movement, then layering nutrition, strength, mobility, and recovery the overall load on the body can become more manageable, making it easier to sustain change.

This approach does not promise quick fixes, dramatic before-and-after images, or guaranteed outcomes. Bodies are diverse, histories are complex, and circumstances vary. What this book offers is an invitation to practice in a way that respects those realities: clear, compassionate rhythms that many people find workable; explanations that aim to be accurate and accessible; and tools you can adapt to your context. It is educational in nature and meant to complement and not replace the guidance of qualified health professionals, especially if you are managing medical conditions.

So take one more gentle breath. Feel the ground beneath your feet the quiet, reliable support that has always been there. Let your exhale lengthen without effort. Then step forward into this journey not by fighting your body, but by partnering with it to be more curious, patient, and willing to return again and again to what helps you feel connected and well.

Welcome to this journey.

Welcome back to yourself.

Start From The End

Picture two endings.

In the first, an older woman sits by a window in the late afternoon light. She moves slowly but on her own. There's a book on the table, a mug she carried from the kitchen, and a phone buzzing with messages from people she loves. She is not perfect like no one is but she is present. She gets up when she wants, walks when she wants, and goes to bed satisfied with a life she can still participate in.

In the second, an older man lies in a bed he rarely leaves. Morning and night are measured by alarms with pills to wake, pills to sleep, pills to soften the side effects of other pills. He depends on someone else to sit him up, to help him to the bathroom, to remember the next appointment. Everyone is trying their best, the family, doctors, nurses but the rhythm of his days is not his own.

Most of us dream of the first ending. We want to live long, yes, but more than that we want to live well with clear-headed, mobile, able to enjoy the people and moments that matter. The hard truth is that many people end up closer to the second ending. Not because of bad luck alone, and not because they "failed" in some moral sense, but because the small choices and environments of adulthood slowly shaped their bodies toward it. That is why we start from the end: to be honest about where our current path points, and to choose a different direction while we still can.

Think of life in three broad phases: Youth, Adulthood, and Elderhood. It's a simple model, not a rule book. For many people, these phases add up to around seventy to eighty years, with big differences between countries and circumstances. What matters here isn't the exact number, but what tends to fill those years. Across the world, people are less likely to die from sudden accidents or infections and more likely to die from long-term conditions like heart disease, stroke, chronic lung problems, cancers, diabetes, dementia, kidney disease. These conditions often arrive with a long runway. They start quietly, build slowly through Adulthood, and then define Elderhood.

Not everyone has a specific diagnosis on the last page of their life. Sometimes the body simply wears down; organs tire, repair slows, systems fail. That's natural. But for many, the final stretch is not peaceful. It is a steady narrowing of life with more medications, more appointments, less strength, less independence. The dignity we all want becomes hard to hold when a day requires help for every basic task. It isn't always the number of years that hurts; it's the quality of the years lost.

If you've watched someone you love in that situation, you know how heavy it can be for a whole family. Breathlessness that makes a short hallway feel like a mountain. The fear after a stroke that it could happen again. The silent weight of a cancer scan. The confusion of dementia moments of clarity mixed with moments where faces blur. The routines of diabetes that never take a day off. Dialysis that rearranges lives. Even when treatments help, the cost in time, energy, and attention is real.

Most of this doesn't begin in Elderhood. It begins in Adulthood. That's the season when we often stop moving, sleep too little, eat on autopilot, and carry stress like a second skin. We tell ourselves it's temporary "just till this deadline," "just till the kids are older," "just till we get through this patch." Then years pass. Somewhere in the middle of doing everything for everyone else, we quietly stop taking care of ourselves. By the time our 50s or 60s arrive, the body is still going, but on fumes. It's trying to survive each day rather than support a life we enjoy.

Why push that hard in the first place? Usually for love and security. We work to provide, to build stability, to give our families choices we never had. We tell ourselves we'll enjoy it "later." But there is a question we can't ignore: what is the use of freedom if our bodies can't come along? If we run so hard in adulthood that we collapse in Elderhood, the people we meant to protect may end up protecting us at a cost to their own lives. That's not anyone's fault. It is, however, a predictable outcome of a culture that rewards urgency and neglects recovery.

Here's the paradox: the fastest way to reach anything meaningful is to slow down. Slow down enough to eat a real meal. Slow down enough to move your body most days. Slow down enough to sleep. Slow down enough to say no to one more obligation that steals your health for free. Slowing down isn't laziness; it's maintenance. It's how you keep the machine that carries you i.e your body—running well enough to enjoy the life you're building.

Many of us make it through Adulthood at all because of what we banked in Youth. Think about it: hours of play, walks and sports, climbing, sunlight, regular bedtimes (even if we didn't like them), mostly simple, home-cooked food. That base can carry a person astonishingly far, even if they neglect it later. But a base only lasts so long. By Elderhood, the bill comes due. And there's a new complication: today's youth is different from the one many of us remember. More screens, less outdoor play. More ultra-processed snacks, fewer shared home meals. Later bedtimes, earlier alarms. None of this makes kids "bad"; it just means their base is often thinner. When the foundation is weaker, Adulthood cracks sooner. We're seeing more people struggle earlier with conditions that used to be associated with later life. The pattern isn't identical everywhere, but the direction is clear enough to take seriously.

This doesn't mean medicine is the enemy. Treatments save lives, reduce symptoms, and extend independence. But taking many medications at once which is known as polypharmacy, is common in later years and can quietly drain quality of life. Side effects pile up. Pills get added to manage the effects of other pills. The calendar is filled with check-ins and tests. The goal in this book isn't to reject medicine; it's to delay and simplify it where possible by building a stronger daily life now.

So why begin a fitness journey at all? Because you are not chasing a number on a scale, instead you are building a healthspan. Lifespan is how long you live. Healthspan is how long you live well: mobile, steady on your feet, able to lift a bag, climb stairs, play on the floor with a child, carry yourself through a busy day without pain screaming for your attention. Fitness is the simplest, most reliable tool we have to protect healthspan. It improves blood sugar control. It strengthens the heart and lungs. It preserves muscle and bone, the very tissues that keep you moving and prevent a small fall from becoming a life-changing event. It sharpens mood and sleep. No pill can do all of that at once.

This isn't about guilt. We live inside systems and habits that nudge us away from caring for ourselves. Cheap, tasty food is available everywhere. Sitting is built into how we work. Stress is normalized and recovery is optional. None of that is your personal failing. The first step back is not blame; it is awareness, seeing how the current makes you drift so you can choose a different line across the water.

Take a clear look at your ordinary day. Where are the small places to turn the wheel? Ten minutes of walking after a meal. An extra glass of water before coffee. A bedtime that protects one more hour of sleep. A packed lunch twice a week. A set of push-ups by the kitchen counter while the kettle boils. These are not grand gestures. They are signals to your future self: "I am building you a better ending."

Starting from the end gives us a test for every choice in Adulthood: Does this move me toward the ending I want? If the answer is no, can I choose a slightly better version today? Not perfect but better. We don't need a complete life renovation to change direction. A few daily changes, repeated, steer the ship over time. That is how most people arrive at the first ending, the one by the window with a book and a mug and enough strength to stand up and get what they need.

If you are thinking, "I already know this," you're probably right. Most of us do. We feel it in the lingering fatigue, the tight chest, the short temper that comes with poor sleep, the voice that whispers, "This isn't sustainable." My job here isn't to surprise you; it's to make the truth you already sense impossible to ignore and simple to act on.

And if you haven't felt that realization yet, stay with me. You might notice it in a parent's slow walk, a friend's lab results, or a moment when you needed help to do something you used to do alone. Awareness arrives at different speeds for different people. When it does, it helps to meet it with kindness, not shame. You are not behind. You are right on time to start.

One more thing about money and time. We often trade health for both, telling ourselves we'll "buy it back" later. But the market doesn't work that way. Money can pay for good care, for guidance, for a safer environment but it cannot buy back lost muscle, lost years of movement, or a heart that has been overworked for decades. The most cost-effective investment you can make is steady attention to your body now. It pays out later in freedom: the freedom to walk, to travel, to play, to live without a schedule ruled by appointments and refills.

None of this guarantees a perfect Elderhood. There are no guarantees in health. Genetics, accidents, and pure chance will always have a say. But that is not an argument to give up. It is a reason to control what you can. Every helpful choice stacks the odds toward the ending you want. Every day you move, sleep, and eat a little better is a day you gain, not just at the end of life but tomorrow morning when you wake up clearer and stronger.

So start here. Start from the end. Pick the ending you want and let it pull you forward. You don't need a gym membership yet. You don't need special gear. You need a decision and the smallest step you are willing to repeat. Walk for ten minutes today. Do it again tomorrow. Choose a real meal once more this week. Go to bed half an hour earlier. Tiny is fine. Tiny builds. Tiny changes your path.

Reclaim your body. Reclaim your energy. Reclaim your life.

Your future self and the people who love you will thank you for choosing a better ending, starting now.

Cutting Through the Noise

Open any app and you'll find a thousand voices telling you what to do: fast this, lift that, don't eat this after 7 p.m., only eat that before noon, drink this to "detox," run more, never run or just walk. No wonder health feels confusing. But underneath all the noise, there's a simple signal worth listening to: a real fitness journey is not a 30-day stunt. It's not a crash diet for a wedding or a two-week sprint before a beach trip. It's not about one photo, one outfit, or one season. It's a way of life.

When I say "fitness," I don't just mean barbells, marathons, or meal plans. I mean the strength, energy, and inner steadiness to move through your day with less effort and more confidence to wake up clear, to climb stairs without gasping, to carry groceries without thinking twice, to handle stress without breaking down, and to meet each day in a body that feels like it's on your side. And when I say "journey," I mean time. Growth. Setbacks. Learning. Progress that sometimes shows up in the mirror, and often shows up in how you feel. A path that unfolds in small steps, repeated.

Most people don't begin this journey with excitement. They begin with discomfort. A lab result that scares them. A flight of stairs that feels longer than it should. A mood that stays flat even on good days. A sigh in front of a mirror that says, “Something is off.” Whatever the trigger, the destination is the same: a life that feels more vibrant, steadier in the mind, and lighter in the body, a life where you don’t just get through the day, you’re present in it.

To get there, we need clarity about what “healthy” actually means. Health is not just the absence of illness. It isn’t simply being pain-free or avoiding diagnosis. True health is a whole-person state physical, mental, and social well-being working together. It’s your heart, lungs, muscles, brain, and immune system doing their jobs; it’s your emotions staying manageable under pressure; it’s your relationships feeling safe, respectful, and real. If any one of those pillars is neglected, the structure wobbles.

We often forget the social pillar. We obsess over steps, macros, or bedtimes and overlook the health of our connections. Yet you can eat well and train hard and still feel empty if your relationships are brittle. Social well-being shows up in ordinary moments: the tone you use with your partner, the patience you have with your children, the time you make for a parent, the way you collaborate with a colleague, the friend you check on without a reason. When this part of life is healthy, you feel emotionally safe around your people. You can speak honestly, listen deeply, and disagree without damage. You feel seen, supported, and like you belong.

When it's frayed, the signs are quiet at first: disconnection in a house that looks busy, a smile that doesn't reach the eyes, a sense of being invisible in a room full of people. That kind of loneliness whispers. Over time it affects the mind; everything feels a bit harder to manage, small triggers feel bigger, fatigue shows up before the day starts. And when the mind is overloaded, the body follows. Workouts slip. Meals are decided by convenience. Sleep shortens. The whole system tilts.

This is why a true fitness journey goes beyond chasing visible changes. Getting "in shape" is only one piece. Real, durable health is alignment: your actions support your mind, your mind supports your relationships, and your relationships support your actions. Each part strengthens or weakens the others. None of this requires perfection. It requires coherence.

Today that coherence is harder to find. Life feels crowded. Notifications tug your attention. Work leaks into evenings. The scroll stretches the night. Even gentle structure breathing for two minutes, sitting still, turning off the light on time can feel heavier than continuing on autopilot. It's not that you don't care about your health. It's that pausing to care feels like one more task on an already full list. So you reach for relief: another episode, another party, another drink, another hour online. These soothe in the moment but don't restore what's empty. They are escapes, not repairs.

When people finally try to "be good," they often pick the hardest version first. They set strict sleep rules they can't follow, cut entire food groups overnight, or punish themselves with long, draining cardio sessions. Then comes guilt when the plan collapses. That's when shortcuts start to sparkle: powders that promise to cleanse, drinks that promise to "detox," hacks that claim to melt fat while you rest. Here's the truth: your body already has a detox system, your liver and kidneys. No tea or cleanse can replace basic habits. Quick fixes are loud. Fundamentals are quiet. But it's the quiet ones that change you.

When the fundamentals are neglected, the body speaks up. Fatigue that coffee can't fix. Sleep that never feels deep. Aches that tag along all day. Mood swings that don't match what's happening. We look outside for miracles for a new supplement, a superfood, a cutting-edge routine all hoping for big change without changing ourselves. But the deeper work is inside: rebuilding the basics.

Part of that rebuilding happens in your brain. The part that helps you plan, resist impulses, and choose long-term gains over short-term relief, the prefrontal cortex, works best when you sleep enough, move regularly, and manage stress. When sleep is cut short and stress is constant, that system gets noisy. Self-control feels costly. Saying no to junk or yes to a walk becomes harder not because you're lazy, but because your brain is operating in survival mode. The good news is the loop runs both ways. Small wins, an early night, a short walk, a balanced meal all make the next good choice easier. Routines are not just behaviors; they're brain support.

If earlier generations didn't talk about "discipline," it's because daily life quietly built it. People woke with the sun, moved through chores, ate simple meals, and slept in darkness. Health was a byproduct of their routine. Many focused first on survival and finances and we inherited that script: "First money, then health." But times have changed. Today's environment invites sitting, snacking, scrolling, and sleeping less. Health is no longer guaranteed by routine; it has to be chosen on purpose. The new script is this: Build both strong finances and strong health, because one without the other limits your life.

And here is a surprising relief: your body is not as complicated as the internet makes it. It feels overwhelming because advice is conflicting and loud. When you understand a few basics and practice them repeatedly, care becomes simpler than you expect. That's what this book is for: not to drown you in rules, but to give you the kind of clarity that turns effort into traction.

So what actually cuts through the noise? Start with the foundations and keep them small enough to repeat:

Move most days, in ways that use your whole body. Think walking, stair-climbing, pushing, pulling, squatting, carrying. Don't chase exhaustion; chase consistency. Movement improves energy, sleep, mood, blood sugar, and the strength of your heart, muscles, and bones. No single pill can do all of that at once.

Eat mostly real food most of the time. Build meals around protein, fiber, and healthy fats. Add color from plants. Keep ultra-processed foods in their place, not forbidden, just not the base of your diet. Don't hunt for magical foods; build reliable meals. If you like rules, keep them kind: add one serving of vegetables, drink one glass of water, include one palm of protein. Simple scales.

Sleep like it matters because it does. Pick a bedtime you can keep most nights. Dim evenings. Defend mornings from your phone for a short while. Treat naps as tools, not escapes. Sleep makes every other habit easier.

Step outside daily. Sunlight sets your body clock, lifts mood, and pairs well with movement. A ten-minute walk after a meal does more for your health than most fancy routines.

Connect on purpose. Don't wait for harmony to arrive by itself. Send the text. Take a walk with a friend. Eat at the table. Ask a real question and listen to the answer. Stronger relationships buffer stress and make healthy routines stick.

Notice the loop: care for the body, and the mind steadies; protect the mind, and relationships mend; strengthen relationships, and daily choices get easier. No single pillar carries everything. Together, they do.

You don't need to prove anything to start. You don't need gear, a program, or a perfect plan. You need a decision and the smallest step you're willing to repeat. Think of these as "signal habits," simple actions that quiet the noise. Ten minutes of walking after dinner. A balanced breakfast you can assemble on autopilot. Lights out half an hour earlier. Two minutes of breathing before you check your phone in the morning. One strength moves while the kettle boils. Tiny is fine. Tiny builds. Tiny changes your path.

Will fitness guarantee perfect health? No. Genetics, luck, and life still have a say. But a fitness journey done the quiet way that shifts the odds in your favor. It lengthens healthspan (the years you live well) and supports lifespan (the years you live), and just as importantly, it changes how tomorrow feels. You wake clearer. You move easier. You show up better for yourself and for the people you love.

I can light the way, but only you can take the steps. Start with one signal habit today. Repeat it tomorrow. Let the results be slow and real. That is how you cut through the noise by building a life that makes sense from the inside out.

Don't Fight, Grow

Picture two starts the same week. On Monday, Gayatri wakes up fueled by a burst of resolve. She writes a strict plan: no sugar ever, 6 a.m. gym every day, perfect eight-hour sleep, tracked meals, meditation, journaling, three liters of water while still nailing work and family. By Wednesday night she's exhausted, behind, and quietly angry with herself. On Thursday, she quits and calls it "lack of willpower." The next Monday, she repeats the cycle.

Now picture a different start. Same Gayatri, same life. She chooses one change: a ten-minute walk after dinner. She puts her shoes by the door and sets a simple cue: "When I put down my plate, I'll walk." That's it. By Friday, the walk feels normal. The next week she adds lights-out thirty minutes earlier, most nights. Over time, the small things stack. She doesn't feel conquered; she feels supported. Nothing dramatic. Everything is different.

Up to now, we've talked about why fitness matters and what it really means. This is where ideas become action. The honest truth is that most people don't "fail" because they're lazy or weak. They're overwhelmed. They're handed the wrong map: an all-or-nothing culture that demands an overnight makeover, cut everything, perfect everything, be someone new by tomorrow and then blame them when it collapses. If that has been your experience, you're not broken. The method is.

Real change isn't a switch you flip; it's a capacity you grow. It's not a fight you win once; it's a relationship you build over time. You don't need to reinvent yourself. You need a daily rhythm that respects your real life. Fitness begins with how you move, how you eat, how you sleep, and how you work with your emotions but the shift happens when those stop feeling like punishment and start feeling like care. A morning walk becomes a way to clear your head. A simple, home-cooked meal feels like nourishment, not restriction. Going to bed on time becomes a way to protect your peace.

The real work happens in moments no one sees. In the breath you take before replying when stress hits. I'm standing to stretch after an hour at the desk. In five minutes of loosening your body before bed. In the pause before you grab your phone to numb out. These are small choices, but they're powerful. Every time you choose awareness over autopilot, you strengthen the inner skill that holds every habit in place.

As awareness grows, you begin to notice which foods leave you steady and which leave you foggy. You feel which routines give you energy and which quietly drain it. You stop chasing health that looks good on a screen and start building health that feels right in your body. This is not about control; it's about connection.

I learned this the long way. For years, I believed grit could solve anything. I coached myself and others like we were machines: push harder, add more, suffer now, reward later. And sure, sometimes that worked, briefly. But over time, life softened my edges. I started listening. Not to rules, but to results I could feel: energy that lasted after a meal, clarity after a walk, calm after better sleep. I stopped trying to dominate my body and started partnering with it. That shift of less force, more awareness all changed how I lived and how I coach. Fitness stopped being a battle to win and became a relationship to tend.

Life isn't tidy. There will be days you miss a workout, nights you sleep badly, moments you eat for comfort, mornings your mind feels scattered. That's not failure; that's being human. The difference isn't in avoiding slips whereas it's in how quickly you return. Strength isn't built by intensity alone, in fact it's built by returning often enough for progress to compound. Consistency turns small actions into big outcomes.

Returning is easier when you meet yourself with respect instead of judgment. Shame freezes action; self-respect restarts it. So when you wobble, trade "I blew it" for "I'm back." Ask a better question: What's the smallest thing I can do next? Drink a glass of water. Take a five-minute walk. Turn down one late-night scroll. Go to bed half an hour earlier. Tiny is fine. Tiny builds.

Make the return automatic with simple "when-then" plans. When I finish dinner, I'll walk ten minutes. When the kettle boils, I'll do ten countertop push-ups. When I plug in my phone at night, I'll set my bedtime alarm. These cues remove the guesswork. They don't require perfect motivation; they ride the routines you already have.

You'll notice something else: the loop runs both ways. Sleep better and your choices feel easier. Move a little and your mood steadies. Eat a balanced meal and cravings quiet down. Protect your mind and your relationships feel safer; strengthen your relationships and healthy routines stick. No single pillar carries it all. Together, they do.

Flexibility matters as much as effort. Rigid rules snap under real life; flexible structure bends and returns. Some days, honoring your body means movement: a walk, a stretch, a workout. Other days, it means rest, real rest, without guilt. Sometimes it's hydration. Sometimes it's turning off your phone and breathing in the quiet. Sometimes it's saying no. Sometimes it's calling a friend. The answer changes because you change your energy, emotions, and circumstances ebb and flow. Let your plan adjust without abandoning it.

If you're at the starting line, begin where you stand. Choose one habit you can repeat even on a busy day. Put it on rails with a cue. Keep the bar low enough that you rarely miss. If it feels too easy, that's good you're building a base you can actually keep. Next week, add one more small thing. That's how rhythms form: not from heroic bursts, but from ordinary actions done often.

Remember why this matters. You're not chasing a perfect body or a flawless routine. You're building a healthspan, years lived well, in a body that lets you do what matters. You're building a mind that can steer when stress rises, and relationships that feel safe enough to hold you while you grow. No routine can guarantee perfect health, but the way you live can tilt the odds toward the life you want and make tomorrow feel better on the way there.

So ask the only question that really guides this chapter: What would honoring my body look like today? Answer it simply. Do that thing. Then come back tomorrow and answer it again. Over time, your answers will become a living rhythm less about rules, more about respect.

Fitness doesn't live in a gym. It lives in your choices when no one's watching: the way you breathe through a hard moment, the way you carry yourself across an ordinary day, the way you return to yourself after a slip. That's not just fitness. That's freedom. And you grow it patiently, quietly; one small, honest step at a time.

Discipline Is a Joy, Not a Jail

Before we go any further, it's worth clearing up a common misunderstanding. In the previous chapter, I emphasized steady effort, adaptable routines, and staying connected to yourself through awareness. That was not an invitation to abandon discipline or to treat consistency as optional. Doing so would undercut long-term progress. In reality, those ideas are expressions of discipline and consistency in their most sustainable form, not the rigid, punishing version often portrayed in popular culture, but a steadier, wiser approach that grows from understanding, awareness, and patience. They are the core scaffolding that allows effort to endure.

What I am saying is this: discipline should not feel like a burden you haul through your days, and consistency should not feel like pressure closing in around you. When built well, these habits strengthen your mindset instead of draining it. Think of them as reliable tools or methods you can reach for rather than rules that rob you of peace. The kind of discipline that lasts is rooted in clarity, purpose, and an honest sense of what matters to you. That inner alignment is what keeps you moving forward, not because you are being forced or frightened into action, but because you have chosen to stay committed.

It helps to step back and examine the cultural messages we receive about effort. We are repeatedly told that “real commitment” equals intensity: dive in headfirst, never pause, never adjust. Slogans like “grind harder,” “no excuses,” and “push through no matter what” get treated as universal truths. If you’re not doing that, the implication goes, you must not be serious. Yet that picture confuses pressure with discipline. Pressure often produces exhaustion rather than resilience, and burnout rather than growth. Discipline, by contrast, is a structure that supports you over time; it adapts when life does, and it holds even when motivation dips.

We also tend to imagine discipline and consistency as inherently extreme like endless self-denial, never missing a day, forcing yourself forward regardless of context. Part of that belief may come from the way we look at people who’ve achieved meaningful results. We see the outcomes and assume the path required extraordinary, almost superhuman sacrifice. Our minds build a story to match the accomplishment: “It must have been brutally hard. Otherwise everyone would do it.” From there, it feels natural to assume discipline is always a monumental, painful struggle. But that story overlooks how the most durable change actually unfolds.

A more realistic account is quieter: many people who sustain strong routines begin with a single, manageable action that fits their current life. They repeat it, adjust it, and make it just challenging enough to stay engaging.

Over time, through patient iteration, that once-small behavior grows into what looks from the outside like an impressive routine. The work is not easy, but it is rarely theatrical. It's a series of ordinary choices made consistently enough to become reliable. The path isn't glamorous; it's cumulative.

Real discipline is not loud. It doesn't rely on extremes or all-or-nothing thinking. It is steady, structured, and purpose-driven. It isn't about doing more every day; it's about doing what matters with intention and control. Useful discipline aligns you with your goals not by frightening you with failure, but by providing direction. It helps you learn when to press and when to pause so you don't break down over the long run. Imagine steering a car with steady hands and not clenching in panic, but guiding with calm awareness, clear about where you're going and why.

And consistency? It isn't about perfect repetition. It's about having something dependable to return to. Think of it as a trustworthy teammate or mentor that is present without nagging, steady without shaming. Consistency reminds you of what you're capable of, especially on the days you forget. That's real accountability: not a spotlight of judgment, but a compass that still points north when enthusiasm fades. This kind of consistency doesn't simply keep you on track; it strengthens your mindset by reinforcing the identity "I'm someone who returns," through intention and long-term commitment.

Here is an image that captures this stance. Picture an artist standing before a blank canvas. In the quiet before the first brushstroke, there's a focused calm, a readiness to begin. The canvas is not a threat or a test; it's an opening, a space where something living might take shape. In that pause, the artist accepts that creation can't be rushed or perfectly scripted. There is uncertainty, but it is held with steady hands and an open heart.

As the work starts, every movement is deliberate yet natural. The brush glides, pauses, and glides again; colors blend and separate; textures appear by gentle layering. Each stroke carries intention, neither hurried nor careless, something like meditation in motion. The artist is not wrestling the canvas into submission or racing toward a finish line. They are immersed in the process itself: the feel of pressure against the bristles, the shift of light across fresh paint, the interplay between control and release. Progress may be slow or uneven, but presence keeps the work alive.

In those moments, the process becomes its own reward. It is not driven primarily by fear of failure or hunger for praise, but by a measured devotion to the act of making. The goal is not to finish flawlessly; the goal is to keep participating, stroke by stroke, even when the improvements are subtle or invisible. Each small choice matters. A single careful stroke can reshape the whole. Meaningful outcomes rarely appear all at once; they reveal themselves as trust deepens and attention remains steady. The painting stops being "just an object" and becomes a record of patience, presence, and skill growing together.

This is what sustainable discipline feels like not a command shouted from the outside, but a calm commitment that rises from within. It’s less a checklist to grind through and more a practice of showing up. Choice by choice, breath by breath, you build something that lasts.

Health and fitness work the same way. You do not need perfection or rigidity to make progress. You need a rhythm of showing up with intention. Adjust when life gets messy. Shift when routines get interrupted. And then return. You are not here to copy a template; you are here to craft an approach that reflects your actual context, values, and constraints. The program that works is the one you can keep doing.

There will be days when you feel strong; clear-headed, focused, full of energy. There will be days when everything feels heavy when you’re tired, distracted, or simply unmotivated. This is not failure; it is a normal fluctuation in human experience influenced by sleep, nutrition, stress, environment, hormones, and countless other factors. Like any craft, real progress includes both forward momentum and slower periods. Some days feel like breakthroughs, others feel like setbacks, but both teach you something useful. Both shape your capacity.

The aim is not perfection; the aim is presence. You are not here to satisfy an impossible standard. You are here to remain involved with your own progress, to notice, to adjust, and to keep returning with direction rather than pressure. When you participate consistently, even imperfectly, you develop resilience. You learn how to continue on ordinary days, not just extraordinary ones. That is the soil in which long-term transformation takes root.

If you're wondering, "Does this mindset actually hold up in real life?," the short answer is yes, and there is a scientific basis for why it often works better than white-knuckle force. Your brain tends to consolidate habits more effectively when behaviors are paired with some sense of internal reward feelings such as satisfaction, meaning, progress, or relief. This is not motivational fluff; it reflects how learning and motivation are shaped in the nervous system.

A brief overview helps. When we repeat an action, networks of neurons coordinate to produce that behavior. Communication at their junctions, synapses becomes more or less efficient over time through processes often grouped under "synaptic plasticity" (including mechanisms like long-term potentiation and long-term depression). Several neuromodulators influence this plasticity. One of them, dopamine plays a well-studied role in reinforcement learning and motivation. Dopamine-releasing neurons in midbrain regions (notably the ventral tegmental area and substantia nigra pars compacta) project to areas such as the striatum and prefrontal cortex. When outcomes are better or more salient than expected, dopamine signals what researchers call a "reward prediction error," which helps the brain tag the events and actions that preceded that outcome as noteworthy. In everyday language, you can think of dopamine as a signal that highlights "this mattered" and makes it more likely that the associated behavior will be repeated.

That signal is content-agnostic: dopamine can reinforce helpful or unhelpful routines alike, depending on what feels rewarding or relieving in the moment. Late nights out, endless scrolling, and certain foods can all be experienced as immediately rewarding, which is partly why those patterns can become sticky. By the same logic, small, meaningful wins like finishing a short walk, completing a set of gentle exercises, or taking a minute to breathe and reset can also acquire staying power when you notice and appreciate them. Over time, repetition with reinforcement strengthens the circuitry that supports the behavior, making the action feel more familiar and accessible.

It's also useful to consider your body's arousal systems. The autonomic nervous system regulates states ranging from "mobilize and respond" to "rest and restore." The sympathetic branch supports energy and action; the parasympathetic branch (often discussed via vagal tone) supports recovery and regulation. Many rewarding experiences are energizing; others feel calm and settling. Both can coexist with dopamine signaling, and both can support learning in different ways. Practices that reliably increase parasympathetic activity like gentle movement, relaxed breathing, unhurried walks, creative play tend to feel lighter and more sustainable for many people. While the connections between specific neuromodulators and autonomic states are complex, a practical takeaway is clear: linking your routines to experiences that you genuinely enjoy or find meaningful helps them persist without relying exclusively on willpower.

Without some felt sense of reward or meaning, behaviors are harder to maintain. You can force repetition for a while, but the brain does not flag the behavior as especially valuable, and other pressures often crowd it out. When even small actions are paired with “this helped” or “this aligns with what matters to me,” the brain is more likely to treat the behavior as worth keeping. In that sense, habits do not just live in your calendar; they leave traces in your nervous system that make future repetitions easier to initiate.

Stress complicates this picture. When you try to build habits primarily from fear, guilt, or the need to prove yourself, you often recruit systems geared toward short-term protection rather than long-term learning. The amygdala and related circuits help detect potential threats; when they signal distress, downstream pathways (including the hypothalamic-pituitary-adrenal axis) increase stress hormones that prepare the body to respond. Short bursts of stress can sometimes sharpen focus, and in certain contexts stress can bias behavior toward automatic, habitual responses. But chronic or intense stress tends to reduce flexible decision-making, sap enjoyment, and make it harder to adapt precisely the skills you need to sustain a routine when life changes. The result often feels heavy and effortful, not because you’re weak, but because your nervous system is prioritizing immediate safety over exploratory learning. Recognizing this is not an excuse; it’s information you can use to design routines that reduce unnecessary strain and preserve bandwidth for change.

This is the rationale behind the approach in this book. It's not just emotionally easier; it's often biologically easier to maintain. When your habits are anchored in purpose and supported by experiences you genuinely value, they're more likely to stick and to evolve as your circumstances change. Individual differences matter; health conditions, medications, sleep, mood, and environment all influence motivation and learning so there is no one-size-fits-all formula. But the general principle is robust: routines tied to meaning, sized to your current capacity, and repeated with compassionate consistency tend to be more durable than routines enforced by constant pressure.

Let's redefine discipline in that light. Discipline is not "never missing a day." It is not pushing through exhaustion solely to tick a box. It is not turning life into a schedule with no room for adjustment. Real discipline is staying committed in ways that are realistic, practical, and built to last. It's returning again and again even when things are uncomfortable, progress is slow, or motivation is low. It is choosing a durable path over a dramatic one. On that path, consistency doesn't press you down; it holds you up. It is the framework that keeps you grounded when life is chaotic. Let consistency be your support system, not your burden. Let discipline feel like forward movement, not punishment. Let it function as a strategy that strengthens you, not a struggle that wears you out.

And when you fall off track, as everyone does, you don't come back because of shame. You come back because you remember why this matters. Your return is not a frantic chase for quick results; it is a recommitment to long-term health, strength, and stability. That clarity turns restarts into part of the plan rather than evidence of failure. Over time, the act of returning becomes one of your defining strengths.

Just as many artists have one piece that carries their story, the work that reflects the effort, experiments, and revisions, your body and mind will carry the imprint of your choices. Major milestones matter, but what shapes you most is the way you kept showing up: day after day, across good stretches and setbacks, through distractions and restarts. You'll see that lasting strength did not come from intensity alone. It came from staying in the process, choosing movement over inertia, order over chaos, and long-term purpose over short-term relief. You did not need to be extreme; you needed to be steady and clear about what mattered.

In the end, that's what real health is made of not only the visible changes, but the mindset that supports them. It's the decision to keep participating in your own growth. It's the patience to build something real at a human pace. It's refusing to give up on yourself when things get hard, and returning again and again to the practices that help you live the kind of life you want.

The Substitute Trap

In the previous chapter, we explored a simple but often overlooked truth: discipline doesn't need to feel like a constant internal battle. It isn't meant to crush you under pressure or drain your joy. When discipline grows from clarity and purpose, when you can name why a path matters to you, it starts to feel supportive rather than punitive. It becomes less about forcing yourself and more about caring for yourself with intention. But even with that understanding, many people still struggle to follow through on the habits they know are helpful. The question is not whether those habits are valuable; we generally know they are. The question is why they remain hard to keep when life gets busy, stressful, or emotionally complicated.

Most of us already know what supports well-being. Deep, steady breathing can help settle the nervous system; nourishing foods contribute to energy and mood; consistent, sufficient sleep supports attention, emotion regulation, and metabolic health; time in nature often reduces perceived stress. None of this is secret. We read about it, we hear about it, and we may have even felt the benefits firsthand. Yet when stress peaks, when anxiety flares, when we feel lonely or depleted we don't always reach for the practices that tend to help in the long run.

Instead, we're pulled toward quick relief: the endless scroll, the snack that's more habit than hunger, another cup of coffee, the extra episode, the cigarette, the drink. It's not that we suddenly doubt the value of a deep breath; it's that, in that moment, we don't fully trust that the slower choice will help us feel better soon enough.

Part of the difficulty is timing. The options that promise immediate comfort usually require very little effort and deliver rapid sensations of novelty or distraction. They offer a quick shift in feeling of no waiting, minimal friction. In contrast, the practices that typically improve well-being breathwork, walking, journaling, adequate hydration, or earlier bedtimes often feel slower. They ask for presence and a small window of patience. In a culture that rewards speed and stimulation, "slow" can be misread as "ineffective." The result is a tug-of-war between what we know and what we reach for, and that tug-of-war quietly erodes consistency.

This isn't a character flaw. It's a predictable feature of how learning and motivation work in the brain. Human behavior is shaped in part by reinforcement learning: we tend to repeat actions that reliably lead to outcomes our nervous system tags as rewarding or relieving. A key neuromodulator here is dopamine. Contrary to popular shortcuts, dopamine is not a "pleasure chemical" in a simple sense; it functions more like a teaching signal. When an outcome is better or more salient than predicted, dopamine neurons fire in a pattern that highlights the events that led to it, particularly within brain circuits that include the striatum and prefrontal cortex. Over time, the brain learns a shorthand: "When I do this, I tend to feel a certain way." This shorthand is content-neutral; it can strengthen helpful routines or unhelpful ones alike.

Consider a common scenario. You feel emotionally overwhelmed and decide to sit quietly for five minutes. Within seconds, thoughts and sensations that were previously masked by activity become more noticeable. That can feel uncomfortable, especially at first, because attention has fewer places to hide. The eventual benefits of the practice of slower breathing, a steadier mood, improved attentional control often arrive after the initial friction. If you instead reach for your phone, novelty, social cues, and variable rewards (likes, messages, unexpected content) deliver fast stimulation. Your nervous system registers many small, immediate payoffs. The long-term cost, reduced focus, postponed emotions that resurface later shows up after the fact, so it exerts less influence on the next choice. In behavioral science, this tendency to favor immediate rewards over delayed ones is sometimes called temporal discounting. It doesn't mean you lack discipline; it means your brain is doing what human brains generally do: prioritizing what changes how you feel right now.

Over time, a discrepancy can form between what your values endorse and what your history of rewards has reinforced. You may "know" that meditation, a walk, or sleep would help, but your nervous system has a thick stack of recent experiences where scrolling or snacking produced quicker relief. When trust is divided, effort is divided. You might meditate, but half of your attention is still evaluating whether checking your phone would have worked faster. You might choose a nourishing meal and still feel pulled toward sugar to complete the feeling of comfort. The result is muted benefit and premature conclusions "See? That didn't help," which further weakened your willingness to return next time. None of this makes you lazy or unmotivated. It means your learning system needs clearer, more consistent signals that the slower path is worth it.

A practical way to shift this is to understand what the "quick fix" is doing and to build a more accurate expectation of the "slow" practice. Many fast comforts supply novelty and intermittent reinforcement patterns known to engage reward circuitry efficiently. Many slower practices begin with a short window of discomfort before the benefits unfold. That does not mean the slower practice "isn't working"; it means the first few minutes are the price of admission. With repetition, the brain updates its prediction model. If you actively notice even small gains, slightly calmer breathing, a brief drop in muscle tension, a few minutes of clearer thinking and you allow yourself to register these improvements, the experience becomes more intrinsically rewarding. In other words, you help your nervous system highlight, "This mattered."

Stress also shapes the picture. When stress rises, the body shifts toward states meant for immediate problem-solving: attention narrows, energy mobilizes, and the brain is biased toward well-rehearsed responses. Short bursts of stress can sometimes sharpen performance, but chronic or intense stress tends to reduce flexibility and self-reflection, two capacities you need to choose a long-term helpful behavior when a short-term option is available. This is one reason supportive routines work best when they are easy to access and require minimal decision-making: a glass of water already on the desk, a mat left out, a short walk built into the transition between tasks. You're not relying only on willpower; you're designing the path of least resistance to the point where you want to go. The research on "decision fatigue" is mixed in detail, but many people do find that simplifying choices reduces friction. The principle is modest and workable: fewer steps make helpful actions easier to start.

Trust, then, is not just a feeling; it's a by-product of repeated, lived experience. When the brain has enough instances where a practice leads to a desired state, it starts to predict that state more confidently. The upfront friction becomes less intimidating because your expectation is calibrated: "I know the first minute may feel noisy, but minute three tends to feel easier." This is how habits shift from negotiations to defaults. You're not merely "being disciplined"; you are accurately remembering what typically happens next and letting that memory carry some of the load.

A useful analogy lives in devotion and ritual. Take prayer, as one example among many reflective practices. People who pray regularly rarely do so because someone is constantly reminding them. They don't wait for perfect conditions. They return because, through experience, they have learned that prayer helps them feel anchored, connected, or peaceful. It doesn't require a daily argument with themselves because trust has replaced negotiation. The practice is no longer weighed against alternatives each morning; it is simply part of who they are. This isn't about performance or perfection. It's about repeated experience teaching the nervous system, "This matters to me, and it tends to help."

That same pattern can be cultivated with foundational self-care. Imagine treating breathwork, movement, nourishing food, hydration, and sleep as non-negotiable forms of care not from rigidity, but from devotion to what reliably supports you. When stress spikes, the first reflex becomes a slow breath rather than a quick escape; when the day fills up, sleep is protected rather than squeezed; when attention scatters, a short walk resets the system. None of this guarantees a particular outcome; bodies are complex, circumstances vary, and health conditions can change the picture but the overall tendency is clear: routines that align with your values and are repeated gently and consistently usually become easier to maintain.

It's also realistic to note why substitutes are so sticky. Many modern products are designed to maximize engagement through novelty, social reward, and personalized content. These features effectively capture attention and deliver frequent, small bursts of stimulation. That design is not a moral failing; it is an engineering choice that happens to intersect with how human reward systems work. Understanding this makes it easier to approach your behavior with compassion. You're not "bad at habits"; you're navigating tools optimized for instant reinforcement. That's precisely why more deliberate, slower practices need a fair chance to prove themselves. They often require a brief period of practice before their benefits feel obvious. Offering them that window is less about willpower and more about giving your nervous system enough evidence to update its predictions.

When you choose the deeper practice over the shortcut even briefly, and even imperfectly you're not just accumulating minutes of meditation or steps walked. You're accumulating instances of "this helped," which is what shifts trust. These small wins matter. Over days and weeks, they build a quiet confidence not only in the habit itself, but in your ability to return to it. That confidence is the foundation of lasting change. It's also self-reinforcing: the more you experience yourself as someone who returns, the less energy it takes to do so again.

A short story makes the point. A man wants to meditate each morning. He believes in its value and has even felt its benefits on days he follows through. Each night he plans to begin with silence. But most mornings, before his feet touch the floor, his hand finds his phone. "Just a minute," he thinks. Messages, updates, headlines ten minutes become thirty, and the morning window closes. He postpones meditation with a promise to try again tomorrow and carries the quiet frustration of a broken intention. His wife, by contrast, wakes and prays. Not out of obligation, but because it is her anchor. She doesn't bargain with herself or compare options. Even when travel disrupts their schedule or the household is busy, she returns to her practice. Not because life is easier for her or because she has superior willpower, but because experience has taught her that this is the way she wants to begin. The difference is not drama; it is trust built from repetition.

This is the turning point the chapter invites: lasting discipline is less about trying harder and more about trusting more fully. It's not the strictness of your schedule that carries you; it's the solidity of your conviction that a given practice is genuinely good for you. When you no longer compare your core practice with a dozen quick alternatives, you reduce the daily negotiation that drains energy. The habit stops feeling like a task to manage and starts feeling like a place you simply return to. Pressure loosens; presence grows.

None of this requires rigidity. In fact, durable routines are usually flexible. There will be weeks when your capacity changes, days when symptoms, responsibilities, or emotions reduce what's possible. Flexibility prevents collapse by allowing for scaled versions of the same intention: one minute of breathing when ten isn't available, a brief stretch when a full workout won't fit, lights out fifteen minutes earlier when eight hours isn't realistic. These "minimum viable" versions protect the identity "I'm someone who returns," while honoring context. Over time, this combination of devotion and flexibility is what makes consistency feel peaceful rather than brittle.

It can also help to close a few "escape hatches" in advance not as punishment, but as design. Placing the phone across the room at night, queuing a short guided practice, setting out water the evening before, or scheduling a brief walk between meetings are small forms of pre-commitment. They don't guarantee success, and they aren't appropriate for every situation, but they often remove just enough friction to help you start. Starting is disproportionally powerful because it gives your nervous system another chance to experience, "This helped," which is how trust grows.

When you approach your practices this way, motivation becomes less central. You don't need to manufacture enthusiasm each morning or fight an internal battle every time. You return to the breath, to the mat, to the walk, to the page because returning is what you do. Some days the benefit is striking; other days it's subtle. Both count. Both teach your brain that this path often leads somewhere steadier than the alternatives.

Think of this as a quiet form of faith not only in any higher power you might believe in, but in your own physiology and capacity to adapt. Faith that a calmer breath can shift your state. Faith that sleep is not a luxury but a biological necessity that supports memory, mood, immunity, and metabolic regulation. Faith that gentle movement can improve circulation and emotional tone, and that nourishing food can steady energy. None of these practices promise specific outcomes for every person, health is individual, and it's wise to seek professional guidance when needed but as a pattern, they tend to make life feel more workable.

You don't need a rigid routine, and you don't need to punish yourself into progress. What you need is a level of trust in one workable path that's high enough to stop chasing a dozen others. When that trust settles in, when a practice stops being a "maybe" and becomes a foundation discipline changes shape. It becomes quieter, clearer, and far less effortful. You're no longer pushing yourself forward so much as letting a reliable structure carry you. The path you've chosen doesn't compete with every shortcut; it holds its own place in your day.

The hardest part is rarely the practice itself. It is the mental negotiation, the delaying, the comparing, the micro-bargains that happen before you begin. Reducing those negotiations, even slightly, frees energy for the actual work of caring for yourself. Then you don't wake up wondering what you'll choose; you already know. That knowing brings a steadier kind of peace.

So you return. Not with drama, but with devotion. Not because you guarantee a specific result, but because the act of returning has become part of who you are. Breath by breath, step by step, page by page, you keep choosing the process that supports you. In that choice, trust gradually replaces pressure. And while no practice is perfect and no life is without disruption, that trust is often enough to keep you moving in the direction you care about gently, consistently, and with a little more grace.

You're Already Disciplined

Here is a perspective that can quietly change how you see your own life: you are already disciplined. Most of us imagine discipline as something reserved for people who wake before dawn to train, track every task, and glide through color-coded calendars. We look at those examples and conclude, "They have discipline; I don't." But discipline is not a rare personality trait handed to a select few. In practical terms, discipline is repeated behavior that persists over time because it feels worthwhile consistency supported by belief, expectation, and experience. By that definition, nearly everyone practices discipline somewhere. You may reach for your phone within seconds of waking, make your coffee the same way every morning, unwind with a show at night even when you planned to sleep early, or pour a drink the moment work ends because it signals closure. Perhaps you always say "yes" to overtime because productivity feels tied to identity. These are not random acts; they are stable routines that you carry out with remarkable reliability. They exist because, on some level, you expect them to help by offering comfort, control, stimulation, or relief. In other words, your capacity for discipline is intact; the question is where it is being directed.

Seeing discipline this way removes the illusion that you are “starting from zero.” You are not learning how to be consistent for the first time; you are learning how to channel consistency toward the outcomes you value most. That reframing matters, because it shifts the conversation from “Do I have discipline?” to “Which behaviors already receive my discipline and are those the ones I want to strengthen?” Habits that don’t serve you long-term often persist not because you lack willpower but because they deliver immediate, predictable rewards. Modern behavioral science describes this with the language of reinforcement learning: when an action reliably leads to a state your brain tags as valuable pleasure, relief, novelty, social connection you are more likely to repeat it. Over time, repetition in stable contexts builds automaticity: behaviors initiated with less deliberation, guided by cues in your environment and routines stored in brain circuits that include the basal ganglia. None of this requires a moral judgment. It simply explains why your “loyalty” to certain patterns can feel effortless while new routines feel uphill at first.

This helps clarify the role of belief. “Discipline follows belief” does not mean wishful thinking magically produces change. It means that when you expect a behavior to help and you have felt it help your nervous system treats the behavior as worth repeating. Expectancy, perceived value, and identity all influence motivation. In psychology, models like expectancy–value theory and self-determination theory describe this:

you sustain effort more easily when you believe an action will work (expectancy), you care about its outcome (value), and the behavior aligns with autonomy, competence, and relatedness (the core needs identified by self-determination theory). When those ingredients are present, you need fewer pep talks because resistance is lower. You are not pushing as much as you are allowing a well-understood choice to unfold.

You can see this in everyday life. Someone who has repeatedly felt calmer after a morning walk will keep walking, even when the weather is uninviting, because experience has taught them that the first ten minutes of effort are followed by a state they value. A person who lifts weights and notices reduced back discomfort and improved daily function will keep training, not to impress anyone, but because the benefits are concrete. Another person who invests monthly in a diversified fund continues through market dips because they have internalized the logic of long-term compounding. And someone who meditates each day often does so because they have experienced even in small ways more mental space afterward. From the outside, this looks like formidable discipline; on the inside, it feels like alignment. The behavior persists because belief and experience have reduced the friction to start.

Prayer offers a parallel from a different domain. People who pray regularly usually do not debate it each morning. They return to the practice because, over time, it has reliably produced states they value: grounding, connection, perspective. The practice becomes part of identity, which matters because identity-based behaviors are sticky. When you see yourself as "someone who returns," the cost of starting again is small; the behavior is less a task and more a way of being. None of this requires a specific belief system. The point is general: consistency becomes easier when repeated experience builds trust.

If everyone is already disciplined in some direction, the practical question becomes: where do you want that discipline to flow? Health is a strong candidate not because it guarantees any particular outcome but because it often supports many others. Sleep quality influences attention, mood, and metabolic regulation. Regular movement benefits cardiovascular fitness, musculoskeletal resilience, and stress reactivity. Nourishing food patterns support energy balance and long-term cardiometabolic risk. Supportive relationships and time in natural environments tend to reduce perceived stress and improve subjective well-being. Individual responses vary, and genetics, environment, social conditions, and health status all matter, so it is wise to avoid one-size-fits-all promises. Still, as a general foundation, health practices often make it easier to learn, work, relate, and recover. Directing your existing capacity for discipline toward these levers is less about heroics and more about alignment.

Understanding why this redirection can feel hard requires a closer look at how the brain updates its expectations. When outcomes exceed what you predicted, midbrain dopamine neurons fire in a pattern sometimes described as a "reward prediction error" signal; this helps tag the actions that preceded the outcome as important. Crucially, this signal is content-agnostic. It can strengthen both helpful and unhelpful routines depending on what was rewarding in the moment. If late-night scrolling repeatedly delivers novelty and social stimulation, your nervous system learns that “this works now,” while the delayed costs (lost sleep, mental clutter) weigh less heavily on future decisions, a well-studied tendency called temporal discounting. By contrast, many health-supporting practices involve a brief window of friction before benefits are felt: the first few minutes of a workout, the initial restlessness of meditation, the early nights of adjusting a sleep schedule. Because the payout is slower, your brain needs a few consistent, salient experiences of “this helped” before it updates its shortcut. That is one reason small, repeatable wins are so powerful: they create enough evidence to shift expectation.

Stress adds another layer. Acute stress can sharpen focus and at times even bias you toward well-learned actions, which is why some people maintain routines during short, challenging bursts. But chronic or intense stress tends to narrow attention and reduce cognitive flexibility, the ability to weigh long-term payoffs against immediate relief. In that state, the easiest available behavior often wins. This is not proof that you lack character; it is physiology doing its job to conserve resources. To work with this reality, it helps to reduce the steps required to start helpful behavior. Environmental design placing the phone across the room at night, leaving a water glass by the bed, queuing a ten-minute walk between meetings, setting out training shoes shrinks the “activation energy.” Implementation intentions (“If it’s 7 p.m., I take a ten-minute walk around the block”) translate a value into a concrete cue–

action link. These are modest tools, but in aggregate they lower dependence on fluctuating motivation.

At the same time, it's worth broadening what "counts." Research on habit formation suggests that automaticity grows with consistent repetition in stable contexts, and that the time course varies widely across behaviors and people. That means a "minimum viable" version of a practice: one minute of breathing when ten is not available, a short mobility sequence on a hectic day, lights out fifteen minutes earlier can protect identity and continuity. You are not aiming for perfection; you are preserving the thread. This matters because each instance of returning is another data point for your nervous system: "This tends to help." Accumulated, such instances become trust, and trust lightens the lift of discipline.

It is also true that we are all disciplined in different directions because our values and constraints differ. Some people prioritize reading because it expands their world. Others invest effort in style, grooming, or creative expression because those choices align inner and outer life. Some are dedicated to sport or training because it delivers stress relief and a sense of capacity. Others pour energy into relationships because connection feels like the heart of a meaningful life. Entertainment can carry discipline, too films, games, or stories may offer restoration or inspiration when thoughtfully chosen. Across these examples, the common thread is not pressure but trust: "This matters to me, and I feel the difference." The invitation here is not to diminish those commitments but to notice that the same devotion can be extended to health in ways that support everything else you care about.

If discipline "follows belief," how do you cultivate belief without forcing it? Start by replacing vague hopes with understandable mechanisms. Learn just enough about why a behavior helps to make its logic feel real to you. For sleep, that might be knowing that consistent timing strengthens your circadian rhythm, which in turn improves sleep efficiency and daytime alertness. For strength training, it could be understanding progressive overload and tissue adaptation: muscles, tendons, and bones respond to gradually increased demands with structural and functional changes. For walking, it might be seeing how low-intensity movement improves mood through a blend of physiology (circulation, autonomic balance) and psychology (context switch, sense of agency). Knowledge is not magic, but it reduces doubt, and less doubt means less internal negotiation every time you begin.

Then make experience with your teacher. Track signals that matter to you not obsessively, just clearly enough to notice trends. Do you fall asleep faster after a wind-down routine? Is your mood steadier on days you walk at lunch? Does your back feel better when you train twice a week? A simple journal or brief notes can surface patterns your memory might overlook. When you recognize that certain actions predictably move you toward how you want to feel, trust grows. This is not an all-or-nothing shift; it is a gradual recalibration. You stop asking, "Will this help?" and start remembering, "This tends to help." That is the moment when discipline begins to feel less like effort and more like flow.

Importantly, none of this erases the reality of unequal starting points. Health conditions, caregiving responsibilities, financial constraints, trauma histories, and systemic factors can complicate what is feasible. In those contexts, compassion and precision matter even more: tailor goals to capacity, seek professional guidance where needed, and measure progress by what is within your control. The aim is not to conform to an ideal but to build routines that are workable for you and supportive of your life as it actually is.

If your past attempts have been uneven, it does not mean you are broken; it often means clarity was missing. Perhaps the plan was mismatched to your schedule, the dose was too high too soon, or the method relied on constant motivation instead of design and identity. The fact that you are still curious enough to read, reflect, and try again is already evidence of discipline. Treat that curiosity with respect. It is the seed from which more skillful routines can grow.

From here, the work is to offer you grounded explanations and workable systems ideas tested in real lives, tempered by research and by the variability that makes us human. The goal is not to sell a shortcut or guarantee a particular outcome, but to give you enough clarity that trust can take root. When the "why" feels real and the "how" feels doable, something shifts internally. You stop spending so much energy negotiating with yourself, and you start spending it participating in your own care. Often, that is the hinge on which lasting change turns.

Skepticism may still be present understandably. Many people have tried programs, apps, or trends that began with enthusiasm and faded under the weight of complexity or life's unpredictability. If a cautious part of you wonders whether this time can be different, you do not have to silence it. You can give that part evidence. Slow down, read with presence, and notice what resonates in your mind and in your body. Experiment at human pace. Keep what works, adapt what doesn't, and let your own experience be the authority that matters most. When a practice fits your context and values and you feel even small, repeatable benefits discipline often stops feeling like a contest of will and starts feeling like the natural next step.

This is what it means to say you are already disciplined. The circuits for repetition, the capacity for devotion, and the ability to return are present in you now. Your task is not to invent them but to aim them. When trust in a chosen path grows grounded in mechanisms you understand and experiences you can feel discipline follows with less friction. You are no longer dragging yourself into routines out of fear or guilt. You are moving in the direction you have decided matters, supported by knowledge, design, and identity. The result is quieter than motivation speeches and more durable than short bursts of intensity. It looks like you, living in alignment with what you value, with enough flexibility to bend when life does and enough steadiness to begin again. And while no approach fits everyone and no routine erases difficulty, this combination of clarity, design, and repeated experience tends, again and again, to turn pressure into trust and effort into a rhythm you can keep.

The Hidden Driver

In the previous chapter, we explored a perspective-shifting truth: everyone is already disciplined in the areas where meaning and value are clear. That quiet consistency shows up in many forms: daily reading, a steady fitness routine, caring for family, a reliable sense of personal style, spiritual practices, or simply keeping up with entertainment. We often don't recognize this as discipline because, once the value of an activity is internalized, the effort feels lighter. When our actions align with what matters to us, they begin to flow with less friction and more ease. This is the state of "effortless consistency" we admire in others and frequently overlook in ourselves.

Yet that understanding raises a harder question: what about the habits we know aren't serving us but still repeat? Why can an evening disappear into a scroll? Why do we stay up too late with one more episode despite wanting better sleep? Why do we skip the workout we fully intended to do? Turning to quick fixes, junk food, distractions, or mindless routines despite knowing they pull us away from the life we want isn't a sign of laziness. It reflects how human behavior often prioritizes immediate relief when we're stressed, tired, or overloaded.

A large part of the answer lies in processes that operate outside deliberate awareness of what many people call the "subconscious" and researchers often describe as automatic or nonconscious systems. This background machinery stores learned associations, emotional memories, and well-practiced responses. It isn't guided by long-term plans or ideals as much as by what has reliably felt safe, comfortable, or relieving in the past. So your reflective, goal-setting mind can say, "I want to use my time better," while your automatic systems nudge you toward familiar comforts that previously took the edge off. That internal tug-of-war explains why change can feel uphill. Sustainable change is not just about goals or new information; it asks us to revisit the emotional learning underneath our habits, the part that has linked scrolling with "stress relief" or a particular snack with "comfort." When we bring awareness to this deeper layer and update those associations, discipline starts to feel less like a fight and more like cooperation.

This chapter is about uncovering what truly drives your actions so discipline can shift from protecting momentary comfort to supporting long-term growth, well-being, and integrity with your values.

Many people assume logic should be enough to change a habit. But the automatic parts of the brain do not respond primarily to charts, data, or motivational quotes; they respond to feeling states and the anticipation of relief or reward. Under stress, our minds tend to favor what soothes us fastest, anything that promises comfort, distraction, or a quick lift in mood. If your nervous system has learned through repetition that checking your phone dampens anxiety for a minute or that certain foods soften a low mood, the impulse to reach for those behaviors can become swift and automatic. This is not a moral failing; it's a learned solution to an uncomfortable state.

You might already know the benefits of sleep, movement, breathwork, time in nature, and nourishing food. Knowledge matters: it sets direction and creates options but knowledge alone rarely rewires automatic responses. Emotional experience does. Until healthier behaviors reliably carry a felt sense of reward calm, satisfaction, pride, connection, relief your automatic systems will keep favoring what has felt rewarding before. In other words, the issue is not a lack of willpower; it's that the reward pathways are still tuned to familiar comforts.

The brain is not only rational; it is exquisitely sensitive to emotion and context. When a behavior helps you feel safer or less distressed, the brain "tags" it as useful. That tag can persist even when the behavior has downsides. As a result, less-than-ideal habits can be stubborn not because they are good in the abstract, but because they once "worked" in a particular moment. One of the brain's core priorities is to protect you from immediate discomfort, which is why quick relief often wins out, especially when you're depleted.

Therefore, the work of change is not to lecture yourself into better choices; it is to help your brain feel the difference. The more you pair desired behaviors with small, genuine, positive experiences, the easier those behaviors become to choose. When movement reliably leaves you clearer or more grounded even for a few minutes your mind starts to predict that benefit. When nourishing food is linked to steadier energy or fewer mid-afternoon crashes, your body learns to trust it. Over time, those updated emotional associations increase the likelihood that you'll reach for the new behavior, not out of pressure, but because it now feels like a good answer to how you want to feel.

Modern habit science offers a useful lens here. A well-known framework describes a loop of cue → routine (response) → reward. A cue—an internal state like stress, a time of day, a place, or even a person triggers a routine, which is the behavior itself. Repetition in stable contexts makes the routine more automatic. The loop is reinforced by the reward, which includes any relief or positive feeling your brain learns to expect. With enough repetitions, cues can launch routines rapidly, sometimes before conscious deliberation. Many researchers also highlight that context and friction matter: we repeat what is easy to start and hard to avoid. The structures that support this learning include the basal ganglia and related networks that encode stimulus-response patterns and are tuned by feedback and prediction errors.

Dopamine, a neurotransmitter often discussed in the context of motivation and learning, plays a central role in marking behaviors as worth repeating. Importantly, dopamine is not simply "pleasure"; it is better understood as signaling salience, expectation, and learning from outcomes. When an activity brings relief or a positive shift, dopamine helps strengthen the association between the cue and the routine. This is why some behaviors become "go-to" responses under stress they've been reinforced. None of this makes change impossible; it simply clarifies why repetition in supportive conditions, paired with immediate, meaningful rewards, is so effective.

Emotion also shapes choice. The "somatic marker" idea popularized by Antonio Damasio suggests that bodily feeling states guide decision-making, especially under uncertainty. While no single theory captures everything, the broad takeaway is consistent: feelings and prior emotional learning influence what we select, often before conscious reasoning finishes weighing in. You might also have heard sweeping claims that "95% of behavior is subconscious." That exact figure is not a settled scientific estimate. Peer-reviewed research typically suggests that a large portion of daily behavior is habitual or automatic, with estimates commonly ranging around half under certain conditions. The precise number varies by context, but the practical point stands: a meaningful share of what we do is driven by learned, automatic processes, especially in familiar environments.

The encouraging counterbalance is neuroplasticity, the brain's capacity to change with experience throughout life. Automatic patterns can be reshaped. They tend to shift most reliably through repetition, context design (making desired behaviors easier and undesired ones harder), and emotionally rewarding experiences that help the new behavior "stick." The automatic systems are not persuaded by shame or self-criticism. They learn through consistent, felt proof that a different choice leads to a better state.

This is where alignment between your "two minds" becomes possible. Your reflective, conscious mind is where intentions, values, and deliberate plans live: "I want to move more," "I want to sleep earlier," "I want steadier energy." Your automatic systems prioritize familiarity and what has helped you feel okay fast. When these systems disagree, we feel friction and often default to the old pattern. Alignment grows when the reflective mind sets a compassionate structure and the automatic systems are taught gently and repeatedly that the new behavior is safe, doable, and rewarding in the moment.

Practically, that looks like shaping conditions and expectations. Keep the first step small enough that it feels safe to start. Pair the behavior with cues that already exist in your day. Reduce friction (for example, placing walking shoes by the door or prepping a simple meal component ahead of time). Add immediate, authentic rewards: notice the calmer breathing after a two-minute pause, the warmer mood after five minutes outside, the clearer thinking after a glass of water and a stretch. Over time, these small wins train your prediction system to expect that the healthier choice will help you feel how you want to feel. You're not forcing compliance; you're building trust with yourself.

Framed this way, the aim of the chapter is not to assign blame for past habits but to explain why they felt so automatic. You have demonstrated discipline all along; it may simply have been directed at what your mind predicted would bring the quickest relief. The scroll after a long day offered distraction. The snack during a low moment offered familiarity. Those patterns were attempts however imperfect to regulate difficult states. Understanding that function allows you to update the strategy without shaming the impulse.

From here, choice becomes more spacious. You do not have to overhaul your life overnight. Begin small and specific: one intentional breath before opening a new tab; a short walk, even around the room; one glass of water before coffee; lights out ten minutes earlier. The power of these acts is not in their grandness but in the feelings they create and repeat. When you treat them as care rather than penance, you lay new tracks. Setbacks will happen. That is not failure; it's part of how learning consolidates. Each return to your next kind choice strengthens the path you want.

Over time, many people notice qualitative shifts. Breathwork stops feeling like a chore and becomes a portable source of steadiness. Movement stops feeling like a tax and becomes a pressure valve. Food shifts from micromanagement to a way of supporting energy and mood. Rest becomes something you respect rather than something you have to "earn." None of this is instant or guaranteed; progress is uneven and depends on personal circumstances, stress loads, access, and health. But with patient repetition, honest feedback, and compassionate adjustments, your internal associations can change. You begin to find comfort in the very behaviors that also support your long-term well-being.

Here's what I believe, grounded in this science and in lived experience: each of us has practiced discipline, even when it showed up as devotion to distraction rather than direction. We were seeking relief with the tools available at the time. Once you see how automatic processes are tuned by emotion and repetition, you gain leverage. You can stop fighting yourself and start teaching your system by experience, not by arguing that caring for yourself is a credible path to feeling better, not just later, but also now.

When that lesson takes root, discipline starts to feel different. It doesn't vanish into pure effortlessness, but the baseline struggle softens. The new choices feel more natural because they carry their own rewards. You are not at the mercy of old loops; you are in a relationship with a learning brain that updates with practice. This book will continue to guide you along that path drawing on research while honoring the messy, beautiful realities of real life. We will explore how the body regulates energy and stress, how habits form and uniform, and how you can rebuild your relationship with movement, food, rest, and mindset in ways that are humane and sustainable. As the emotional rewards of those choices accumulate, calmer mornings, steadier afternoons, kinder self-talk, your belief in them deepens.

From there, discipline often begins to feel less like something you must chase and more like a rhythm you can join, a rhythm supported by evidence, shaped by compassion, and reinforced by the everyday proof that your choices help you feel the way you want to live.

Ancient Wisdom

In the last chapter, we explored a liberating shift in perspective: discipline is not primarily a contest of willpower against temptation. It is the natural outcome of emotional belief of what happens when the part of the mind that can explain a choice and the part that actually initiates action begin to agree. When the body and nervous system register a behavior as safe, useful, and meaningful, consistency stops feeling like a fight. It becomes a rhythm we return to with less friction and more ease. This idea can sound modern, yet it echoes insights preserved in older traditions.

This idea is not new. Long before terms like “dopamine,” “habit loops,” or “neuroplasticity” entered everyday conversation, Indian philosophical and educational traditions took seriously the relationship between knowledge and lived experience. The historical Gurukul system did not reduce learning to memorization or compliance. Rather, it aimed to cultivate the whole person's clarity of thought, steadiness of attention, ethical grounding, and a sense of purpose so that what was learned could be absorbed, tested, and integrated. Teachers worked to align understanding with felt meaning, fostering an inner posture from which disciplined action could arise more reliably. What contemporary research now examines in laboratories how repeated actions become easier to initiate, how emotions shape motivation, how attention and memory are trained was approached, in a different vocabulary, as a matter of practice, context, and character.

Modern science uses specific mechanisms to describe these experiences. Dopamine, for instance, is a neuromodulator that helps the brain learn which actions predict rewarding outcomes; it is not "pleasure" itself, nor is it a universal switch for motivation. Habit formation involves networks that include the basal ganglia and is shaped by cues, actions, and consequences; early popularizations call this a "habit loop," which is a helpful model so long as we remember that real behavior is influenced by many factors: context, stress, sleep, emotion, and goals. Neuroplasticity refers to the brain's capacity to change with experience across the lifespan, a process that typically unfolds gradually as repeated practice and meaningful feedback strengthen certain pathways. These explanations do not diminish older wisdom; they help us understand, in different terms, why patient practice and emotionally grounded learning feel so effective.

The point is not merely historical. It is enduring. If our aim is to live with steadier follow-through, it helps to build the inner conditions that make good choices feel safe, familiar, and worthwhile. In that sense, stepping forward can also be a return to a way of learning rooted in trust, clarity, and presence.

Accounts of the Gurukul emphasize a relationship between teacher and student that was less about external pressure and more about patient guidance. A guru was expected to transmit knowledge and to draw out understanding to help a student see why a principle matters, how it fits within a larger life, and how it can be practiced without anxiety or haste. The process used dialogue, reflection, demonstration, repetition, and service. The emphasis fell not only on "what to do," but on discovering an inner "why" strong enough to sustain practice when novelty faded.

This kind of education recognized that repeated exposure paired with meaning changes how effort is felt. In contemporary terms, when a behavior becomes linked to personally significant outcomes: calm, competence, connection, purpose its initiation recruits fewer deliberative resources and depends less on fleeting motivation. Trust in the process grows through experience: small successes, noticed and reflected on, become evidence that the practice is worthwhile. Over time, this reduces uncertainty, and reduced uncertainty often reduces avoidance. The result is not obedience for its own sake, but a steadier ability to choose what aligns with one's values.

The discipline that emerges from such a context is not harsh. It is reverent. It is less about rules than about realization less about being pushed than about being drawn. The tone is quiet and dependable rather than dramatic; it encourages consistency without exhausting the will.

In traditional accounts, a day might begin before sunrise with stillness, movement, study, service, and contemplation. These were not imposed merely as duties; they were practices chosen and explained because they reliably shaped attention, energy, and mood. In modern language, early light exposure can help set circadian rhythms; intentional silence can reduce external inputs long enough for attention to stabilize; movement can modulate arousal and improve cognitive flexibility; meditation and reflective practices can train awareness and reduce reactivity for many people. Effects vary by individual and context, and they accumulate with repetition rather than arriving all at once. Yet the common thread is clear: when a person understands the purpose of a practice and can feel its benefits even subtly, the practice begins to carry itself.

This is the heart of inner alignment. It is not a mystical switch; it is the gradual convergence of belief, experience, and identity. The conscious mind can name the value; the more automatic systems of behavior the routines that run when we are tired, busy, or stressed learn through felt experience that the behavior is safe and helpful. Over time, the practice is less a task and more a part of how one moves through the day. What once required frequent negotiation begins to feel like a familiar support.

Many people today are rebuilding this alignment. When we say we want to rise earlier, eat more thoughtfully, move regularly, or practice mindfulness, the work is not merely to select a technique, it is to help the body and emotions trust that the technique is worth repeating.

When that trust takes root, discipline begins to look less like forcing and more like devotion: not in a narrow religious sense, but as a steady, heartfelt commitment to what helps life flourish.

Our difficulty is rarely a lack of intelligence, morality, or intention. More often, it is a mismatch between the timeline of meaningful change and the speed promised by quick fixes. Modern culture rewards intensity and rapid results, so we default to short challenges and sweeping resolutions. Those approaches can spark momentum, but they often leave out the slower process by which the nervous system learns to favor a new behavior over an old one. Without enough repetition that feels safe and relevant, our automatic responses lean toward the familiar, especially when we are stressed or depleted.

It can help to clarify terms here. People commonly speak of the "subconscious" as the hidden driver of behavior. In research settings, it is more common to distinguish between deliberative, effortful processes and faster, more automatic ones. Neither system is "in charge" all the time; they trade off based on context, energy, and cues. A large share of everyday actions such as how we reach for the phone, how we settle into the couch, how we begin the morning are guided by automatic tendencies shaped by past repetition and emotion. Estimates of how much vary widely and are imprecise; what matters for change is that automatic responses are powerful, especially under pressure, and they can be reshaped through consistent, meaningful practice.

When a new routine is launched with high expectations but little experiential grounding, the automatic system has no reason to prefer it yet. It does not "believe" in the human sense, but it has not learned the pattern. The remedy is neither self-blame nor a harder push; it is the deliberate creation of conditions in which the behavior can be practiced at a tolerable difficulty, paired with experiences that make its value felt, and repeated often enough to become easier to initiate.

We may not live in ashrams or study beside a single teacher, but we can recreate the essential conditions that make learning and discipline gentler: a clear intention, a tolerable starting point, repetition that respects recovery, and reflection that highlights benefits. In the absence of an external guru, your attention can serve as a guide. Your home, commute, or workspace can become a modest Gurukul place where cues are designed thoughtfully and practices are scaled to your reality.

You do not need rigid timetables to begin. What helps most is a reason that matters to you and a practice small enough to repeat even on ordinary days. Motivation will rise and fall; meaning is steadier. When the conscious mind can say, "This helps me think more clearly," and the automatic system has felt that clarity enough times to expect it, resistance often softens. The goal is not a flawless streak; it is a relationship with practice that is respectful and sustainable.

Let your health journey reflect this older wisdom in modern form. Treat it less like a checklist and more like a craft. Explore sleep, movement, breath, and nourishment with curiosity rather than urgency. Notice what changes attention, mood, patience, energy and give those changes language. Language helps memory; memory helps repetition. As trust builds, the practices become easier to keep. The result is not effortlessness in every circumstance, life will still bring stress and change but a greater likelihood that you return to what steadies you.

Many of us long to feel more consistent to make choices that echo our values even when days are full. That consistency does not usually come from turning up the pressure. It grows from intimacy: understanding how a habit feels in your body, how it shapes your thinking, how it fits your hours, and how it supports the person you are becoming. The brain rewires in response to experience and attention, and both are within reach. You do not need extreme protocols; you need practices that are honest, meaningful, and repeatable in your context.

The Gurukul tradition intuited this: that discipline grounded in understanding and care endures more reliably than discipline grounded in fear. Contemporary research adds details about learning, prediction, attention, and stress. Put together, they point to a compassionate approach: go small enough to succeed, repeat often enough to learn, reflect enough to feel why it matters, and adjust enough to keep it humane. Over weeks and months, this becomes a rhythm rather than a trial.

That is the offer of this book: not a rulebook heavy with demands, but a way of working with yourself that replaces force with flow, anxiety with self-trust, and confusion with calm. We will move gently, honestly, and thoroughly one step, one breath, one practice at a time. In the chapters ahead, we will walk together through choices you can test in your own life, paying close attention to what is helpful for you. No promises of instant transformation, only the steady companionship of sound principles, thoughtful experiments, and patient repetition. With time, the distance between intention and action can shorten, and the life you are practicing can become the life you are living.

The Science of Enlightenment

In the deep silence of the Himalayas, far from the noise, speed, and stimulation of our modern lives, there live individuals who seem untouched by time. They are the sadhus, spiritual seekers, ascetics, and yogis who have consciously stepped away from the chaos of daily existence. Not out of rejection or bitterness, but to explore something far more intimate and infinite. Since childhood, we've seen glimpses of them men draped in saffron robes, meditating in icy caves or dense forests, walking barefoot across scorching earth, living on a few sips of water and moments of stillness. To the average person, their lifestyle seems alien. Mysterious. Incomprehensible. How can someone sit still for hours without moving? How can someone go days without food or speak no words for months at a time? When you look more closely when you remove the lens of myth or spiritual fantasy you begin to see something profoundly human beneath their silence. The path of the sadhu is not escapism. It is not a rejection of life, but an immersion into its most essential elements. It is a journey inward, a disciplined, intimate exploration of the most fundamental forces that shape our experience: the body, the mind, the breath, and the emotions. Every fast observed, every mantra repeated, every measured breath has a purpose. It is not performance; it is practice. They are not trying to impress the world. They are trying to understand their own.

In our age, we often chase peace through productivity and search for stillness through more stimulation. The sadhu's way can look extreme, yet it holds up a mirror. It reminds us that genuine transformation does not always require addition. Often it asks for subtraction, less noise, less rush, less internal resistance. We use the word enlightenment to describe what they seek, a term wrapped in gold and mystery, lifted so high it can feel unreachable. But what do we mean by enlightenment when we place it back on the ground and examine it with care? If we peel away the symbolism and look not upward but inward, we find that the answer is not floating in clouds. It is anchored in physiology and behavior. It touches systems that regulate attention, stress, mood, and connection. At its most grounded, enlightenment can be understood as a capacity: a regulated body, a clear and flexible mind, and a heart that can remain open without being overwhelmed. The language is lofty; the mechanisms are earthly.

The human body is always regulating itself in response to the world, and a key player in that regulation is the autonomic nervous system. This network operates largely outside conscious awareness and continuously adjusts heart rate, blood pressure, digestion, pupil size, and countless other processes. Two primary branches, the sympathetic and the parasympathetic, work together in a dynamic balance. The sympathetic branch helps mobilize us for action: it increases heart rate, shunts blood to muscles, and heightens vigilance. The parasympathetic branch helps us recover and restore: it slows the heart, supports digestion, and allows for bodily repair. Although people often talk about these branches like an on/off switch, biology rarely behaves in absolutes. Both systems can be active to different degrees at the same time, and they can alternate rapidly depending on context. Alongside the autonomic system, the hypothalamic-pituitary-adrenal (HPA) axis releases hormones such as cortisol that influence energy availability, immune function, and inflammation. Together, these systems help the body meet the moment.

When the brain detects threats through immediate sensory input, remembered patterns, or even imagined scenarios it can shift toward a mobilized state commonly called "fight or flight." In this mode, sympathetic activity and stress hormones help us respond quickly: heart rate rises, breathing becomes shallow and fast, digestion slows, and attention narrows to potential danger. This response is adaptive and lifesaving. It prioritizes survival in the short term. Yet if mobilization becomes frequent or prolonged, the costs accumulate. The body's longer-term priorities tissue repair, deep sleep, immune balance, fertility, and learning can be crowded out by constant urgency. Scientists sometimes refer to this wear and tear as allostatic load: the strain of repeated adjustment to stressors. It does not mean stress is inherently harmful; challenges can also build resilience but it reminds us that recovery matters as much as effort.

On the other end of the spectrum is a state many people describe as "rest and digest," where parasympathetic processes are more prominent. In this calmer landscape, the heart settles, breathing deepens, the gut resumes its complex work, and the mind can broaden its focus. This is not a special mystical mode; it is a set of conditions that support repair, learning, connection, and creativity. It does not demand complete external safety; life rarely offers that but it benefits from cues of relative safety: steady breath, predictable rhythms, supportive relationships, and environments that reduce unnecessary alarm. In this terrain, sleep consolidates, tissues rebuild, and the immune system can recalibrate. Over hours and days, this quieter biology supports clarity and steadiness. Importantly, calm does not mean passivity. The nervous system functions best when it can fluidly move between mobilization and restoration, matching energy to circumstance and then returning to baseline.

The key insight, then, is not that one state is "good" and the other "bad," but that health depends on appropriate transitions and proportional responses. Extended periods of intense mobilization without recovery can be depleting; so can long periods of under stimulation and disuse. Muscles need load to remain strong; minds need novelty and meaning to stay engaged. Bodies also need signals that say, "you can soften now." The sweet spot is rhythmic balance: periods of challenge followed by periods of repair. Athletes recognize it in training cycles; musicians feel it in phrasing and rest. The nervous system learns in the same way through oscillation.

This lens helps us appreciate the quiet power of the sadhu's practice. From the outside, their conditions appear harsh: fasting, cold, silence, solitude. These are precisely the circumstances that could trigger strong stress responses in many people. Yet some practitioners display a steadiness that seems to contradict the setting. While research on such specific traditions is limited, studies of long-term breathwork and meditation show patterns that point to possible mechanisms: slower resting heart rates in some practitioners, increased heart rate variability (a marker associated with flexible autonomic control), changes in attention networks that make it easier to notice sensations without reflexively reacting, and altered appraisal of discomfort. None of this implies invulnerability, and effects vary widely between individuals. It does suggest that training attention, breathing, and interpretation can reshape how the body responds to challenges.

Consider the breath. Slow, gentle, nasal breathing with a longer exhale can engage pathways that influence the vagus nerve, which helps coordinate parasympathetic activity. Over time, consistent practices like diaphragmatic breathing, mindfulness meditation, and certain forms of chanting may increase the nervous system's capacity to downshift after activation. Psychological skills matter, too. When people learn to observe sensations and thoughts without immediately resisting them, the brain's alarm circuits can quiet more quickly. This is not about suppressing pain or denying hardship; it is about reducing the additional stress created by the story "this must not be happening."

Reframing stress as challenge, cultivating acceptance, and sustaining attention on the present moment are learnable skills that can decrease unnecessary physiological arousal. In that sense, the sadhu in cold wind is not "comfortable" so much as "less threatened by discomfort," and that distinction opens space for composure.

Seen through this grounded lens, enlightenment does not require floating above reality. It looks more like mastery of response. The body may encounter signals that once triggered alarm hunger, cold, uncertainty but the mind and breath send countervailing messages of steadiness. The organism still mobilizes when needed, yet it returns to balance more quickly and with less friction. This is resilience as a skill, not a promise. It emerges from practice, not from pretending we are beyond human limits. It also has boundaries: extreme fasting, breath retention, or exposure practices can be risky and are not necessary for growth. Many of the benefits associated with contemplative training appear with simpler, safer routines applied consistently: regular sleep, moderate movement, supportive relationships, mindful attention, and daily breath practice.

This brings us to a useful working definition. Enlightenment, stripped of mystique and laid alongside science, can be framed as an uncommon capacity for nonreactive presence: the ability to experience life including challenge without being dominated by reflexive resistance. It is not the absence of stressors; it is a refined relationship to them. The sadhu is not free from cold, hunger, or uncertainty. He is freer from the cascade of secondary struggle panic, clenching, catastrophic thinking that often follows. From that freedom, energy that was once spent fighting reality can be redirected into clarity, compassion, and wise action. The biology here is straightforward: fewer false alarms, more timely recovery, better allocation of bodily resources to what restores and repairs.

If we were to translate this idea into a simple equation, we might start with how the body leans toward survival when challenge meets resistance. Challenge can be physical effort, social conflict, or internal pressure; resistance is the mental and physiological bracing that says “no” to what is already occurring. When the two combine, stress amplifies. Attention narrows, muscles tighten, breathing lifts into the chest, and the HPA axis prepares for battle. Some of this is helpful. We need speed to cross the road but when resistance becomes a habit, threat signals arrive even when no action is required. In contrast, growth is not the absence of challenge. It is a challenge paired with acceptance and skillful engagement. Acceptance does not mean passivity. It means meeting what is present without adding extra struggle, then choosing a response. Biologically, that looks like steadier breathing, a heart that can both accelerate and slow as needed, and a mind that can zoom in and out. Psychologists call this psychological flexibility, and it correlates with better coping and well-being across many contexts.

From here, the sadhu’s lesson becomes practical. He does not require perfect conditions to be at peace because peace, for him, is not the same as comfort.

Peace is the ability to maintain a regulated inner life in imperfect conditions. This is why his energy does not leak into constant vigilance. This is why his focus feels unforced. This is why recovery can happen even in simplicity. When signals of basic safety, steady breath, coherent attention, supportive beliefs are strong enough, the body can keep repairing in the background while life unfolds in the foreground. That repair is not instant or guaranteed; it is gradual, like a muscle strengthening with repeated cycles of effort and rest. Over time, the nervous system learns that discomfort is information, not an emergency, and the mind learns it can be with what it feels without being consumed.

None of this needs to be wrapped in promises of miraculous transformation. The evidence from contemplative science is encouraging and nuanced: many people who practice consistently experience reductions in perceived stress, improvements in mood, and changes in attention and self-regulation. Not everyone responds the same way, and outcomes depend on the method, the teacher, personal history, health status, and environment. Extreme practices should be approached cautiously, especially by those with medical conditions. The point is not to imitate a monk's hardships. It is to understand the principles oscillation between challenge and recovery, nonreactive awareness, skillful breathing and apply them in a sustainable way.

So, what does enlightenment mean within this careful frame? It is the cultivated ability to remain grounded when the ground shifts, to let the body mobilize without the mind catastrophizing, and to return to balance without unnecessary delay. It is the art of walking through fire with water in the breath not because fire does not burn, but because panic is not holding the match. It is deeply human: we hurt, we heal, we learn, we fall, we rise. We still feel the weather of life, but we are less likely to be thrown by every gust. In that stability, discipline softens into devotion, and stillness reveals its strength.

In the chapters ahead, we will examine how modern life can keep many of us leaning toward mobilization, constant alerts, unending tasks, sleep debt, processed stimulation and how that tilt leaves the body tense, the mind tired, and recovery delayed. From that understanding, we will begin the practical work of returning slowly, wisely, and consistently to a rhythm that supports growth. We will look at simple, evidence-informed practices that help the nervous system rebalance, clarify how to use challenge without being consumed by it, and explore how to build inner safety that does not depend on perfect outer conditions. Not to promise a life without storms, but to practice the kind of seamanship that makes crossing possible. The growth that lasts. The growth that heals. The growth that frees you.

Rituals that Repair

In the last chapter, we explored the science of enlightenment not as something mythical or unreachable, but as a learnable capacity to regulate the body and mind across two broad physiological tendencies. For clarity, I'll keep calling them Survival Mode and Growth Mode, while also noting what science observes underneath those names. "Survival Mode" usually reflects a coordinated stress response involving the sympathetic branch of the autonomic nervous system and the HPA axis (hypothalamus–pituitary–adrenal), which mobilize energy and sharpen vigilance. "Growth Mode" describes conditions in which parasympathetic activity, especially vagal pathways has more influence, supporting rest, digestion, tissue repair, and social engagement. These are not on/off switches; they are dynamic, overlapping systems that rise and fall throughout the day. What the sadhus, those ancient seekers who walk barefoot through forests and sit in meditation in the Himalayas appear to cultivate, over years and sometimes decades, is not a permanent escape from stress, but flexibility: the ability to let arousal rise when needed and then restore calm quickly, to keep attention steady and the breath rhythmical even in circumstances that would usually provoke reactivity.

Their power doesn't come from white-knuckle force. It doesn't come from the kind of brittle willpower we often glorify. It comes from alignment: practices that condition a nervous system to find steadiness in chaos, a breath that remains slow enough to signal safety, and a mind that can stay open, even soft, when discomfort appears. This is not a miracle. It is a form of mastery, built slowly, patiently, and consciously.

And so a doorway opens for all of us: How are they able to stay so disciplined, so consistent, and so committed for years, sometimes a lifetime, without breaking down, burning out, or quitting? From the outside, it looks impossible. The question is worth asking carefully, because the answer isn't a single trick. It is a web of meaning, biology, attention, and community that, woven together over time, makes consistency feel natural instead of punishing.

To the average person navigating modern life, the daily rhythm of a sadhu can look like pure hardship: fasting for days, meditating for hours in stillness, walking barefoot over sharp stones and cold soil, sleeping little, speaking less, praying from before sunrise until well after sunset. How can that be sustainable? How could that be joyful? A scientific lens doesn't deny the difficulty; it simply notices mechanisms that make difficulty more livable. Extended stillness trains attentional control and interoceptive awareness (the felt sense of the body). Slow, nasal breathing, often around five to six breaths per minute in many contemplative traditions, tends to increase heart-rate variability, a commonly used proxy for parasympathetic influence.

Repeated exposure to manageable discomfort, paired with a sense of purpose and skilled regulation, can reduce threat perception over time. None of this guarantees that a practice is right for every person or circumstance, but it helps explain why some people find such rhythms not only tolerable, but deeply nourishing.

Yet they do not just survive it they often thrive within it. What looks like discipline from the outside is devotion from the inside. What seems like suffering to an untrained mind can feel like freedom to a trained nervous system. They are not driven by pressure; they are moved by purpose. They are not trapped in routines; they are in relationship with them. That relationship changes everything. In neurobehavioral terms, their practices have high “incentive salience”, they feel rewarding, not merely obligatory. Meaning saturates the action. Through repetition, those actions migrate from effortful, top-down control (heavy prefrontal involvement) to more automatic pathways (striatal habit circuits). The result is that consistency stops requiring constant negotiation. It is not born of punishment or fear; it is supported by emotional clarity, deep trust, and an ability to perceive and savor the small, intrinsic rewards of each ritual: calmer breath, steadier mood, clearer attention, a felt sense of alignment.

We forget a simple truth when we rush to “be better” and “do more”: discipline must not feel like punishment if it is to endure. If it feels like self-torture, it will collapse under its own weight. Sustainable discipline, the kind that quietly reshapes a life over years is not built on guilt, force, or fear. It is built on conditions that the body can maintain: predictability, recoverability, and meaning. In research language, this looks like reducing allostatic load (the wear and tear of chronic stress), increasing perceived control, and attaching behavior to values that matter personally. When those ingredients are present, discipline becomes a stable pattern rather than a short-term push. Otherwise, we are just trying to follow instructions we do not believe in, and the brain's natural resistance to coercion eventually outcompetes the plan.

Return to the sadhus. Yes, they fast. Yes, they live without modern comforts. But they move through these routines with an ease, even a quiet joy, that doesn't mean the routines are easy; it means the routines are integrated. Their subconscious associations are aligned with their actions. They don't just know, abstractly, that meditation can calm arousal or that fasting can alter metabolism; they feel the effects in their bones. Over time, the mind and heart learn to agree. Faith no longer lives only in thought; it shows up in breath, muscle tone, and daily choices. The pleasure and relief many people feel while eating comfort food or scrolling a phone are, for them, embedded in silence, mantra, service, and restraint. Mechanistically, repeated pairing of a practice with felt benefits reshapes expectations and prediction signals in the brain's reward circuits, which is why what looks extreme from the outside can become natural from the inside. Consistency then doesn't require a "grind." Bracing gives way to presence. They are not at war with themselves. That is the secret. That is alignment.

In my own life, I grew up inside a family steeped in spiritual values. As a child I followed rules and rituals: prayers, gestures of respect, patterns of devotion that matched our tradition. As I grew older, my belief in God, spirituality, and religion began to fade. I couldn't connect with them; I suspected there was no God at all, and that our practices were inventions designed to control people. With time, though, I realized I had missed something important. The things we do in the name of religion, the rituals and the prayers, are not necessarily about appeasing an external power. Many of them function as behavioral technologies shaped by culture and refined by experience. They organize attention, synchronize communities, anchor habits to meaning, and structure times of stimulation and times of rest. They can support mental steadiness, physical rhythms, and social health. This does not make them magic, and it does not mean every ritual helps every person; it simply means there is often a logic beneath the symbolism.

By the time I understood that, I had already drifted from God as something "out there." What I learned, and continue to learn, is that the presence I was searching for can also be understood "in here." Everything we do in the name of God or spirituality can serve a second purpose: to help us notice that the qualities we long for peace, courage, compassion already have footholds within us, waiting for a relationship. When a practice helps me contact that inner steadiness even briefly, I change how I meet the world.

These practices, then, help us connect with an "inner God," which you can read as your deepest values, the quiet witness, or the soulful core that persists beneath mood and circumstance. In practical terms, connection looks like better stress recovery, clearer priorities, and relationships that feel less brittle. There is evidence that consistent contemplative practice can improve attention and emotion regulation; that shared ritual can strengthen social bonds; that routine behaviors scaffold circadian timing, digestion, and sleep. No single practice guarantees any single outcome, and context always matters, but together these patterns can nudge the system toward resilience.

Today many of us are perpetually searching, waiting for the "right" time, place, person, or perfect moment to feel joy. We keep searching because joy feels disconnected from our daily sensations. Even on busy or productive days, we can end in heaviness. Some people begin wishing life would pass faster simply because they are not enjoying their lives as lived. Stress, anxiety, and emotional pain accumulate. Nearly every religion offers an image of God: a face for the presence already within. In psychological terms, such images serve as attentional anchors and meaning-encoding symbols. They help us focus, they invite qualities (like courage, tenderness, steadiness) into awareness, and they reduce decision fatigue by giving the mind a stable referent.

That is why many sadhus follow one form Shiva, Krishna, Hanuman, Durga, and others. In my tradition of Hinduism, there are many deities; I speak of it because I know it best, while recognizing that other religions use different symbols to point toward similar states. The goal is the same. No one deity is "stronger." What matters is how the image is received in the nervous system, how it evokes emotional safety, awe, gratitude, humility and how that internal response becomes a mirror that reflects what already lives within us.

When we connect with the inner God when we connect with ourselves what once felt impossible becomes comparatively more workable. With emotion, trust, and clarity, consistency gets lighter. Motivation spikes are no longer the engine; meaning is. People who wake early for a picnic do so for a few days because novelty is energizing, and then the brain habituates. People who wake early for spiritual reasons may sustain it for decades, not because they are superhuman, but because the action is tethered to identity and purpose. This is the difference between behaviors fueled mainly by external reward and those supported by intrinsic value. It is also why such practices often spill over into kindness; when internal strain decreases, there is more bandwidth for care.

From here on, the practices I suggest are not religious rituals, though you may recognize echoes of them. I invite you to approach them with the same depth you might bring to spirituality. Don't do them only to "achieve" something quickly; that mindset tends to fade and can backfire. Do them as a way of cultivating relationships with breath, with attention, with your body, with your days. Anchor them in emotional connection, clarity, and, if the word fits you, faith. Also anchor them in prudence: adapt to your body, your medical realities, and your season of life. If you live with a medical condition, are pregnant, or have a history that makes fasting or intense practices risky, seek appropriate guidance. The spirit of the work is gentleness directed with purpose.

Sadhus did not step away from the world to escape; many stepped away to repair. Living in near-constant Survival Mode carries costs: irritability, digestive disruption, sleep disturbance, and, over time, what researchers call allostatic load, the cumulative strain of repeated stress responses. Chronic, unbuffered stress is associated with changes in immune signaling, shifts in hormone patterns, and a greater risk of burnout and several stress-related illnesses. None of these outcomes is caused by stress alone; genetics, environment, nutrition, movement, relationships, and access to care matter. Still, giving the body reliable seasons of safety allows restorative processes to do their quiet work.

Only after years of such repair do some sadhus seem to "hold both modes", to maintain steady breath and attention in conditions that would normally trigger collapse or panic. This capacity is sometimes called stress resilience. It doesn't mean they feel no pain or fear; it means they can sense activation rising, meet it with skill, and re-establish equilibrium more quickly. They, too, had to live separately in both states before integrating them. They had to relearn safety before they could move freely inside stress.

Here is your hope: you do not have to leave your life to heal. You do not need a cave, a robe, or a vow of silence. You need a window small, consistent, and yours. Devoting even 3–6% of your day about 30 to 60 minutes to practices that signal safety and presence can begin to recalibrate your system. This might include unhurried breathing, quiet sitting, a slow walk in nature, prayer or mantra, gentle mobility, mindful tea, sunlight in the morning, or a screen-free hour before bed. Research across different domains suggests that brief daily practice can produce measurable shifts in mood, attention, and physiological markers for many people; your mileage will vary, and that is normal. What matters most is repetition that your body can trust.

There is no shortcut. No hack replaces presence. We can try to trick the body or sprint our way to calm, but the body responds more consistently to cues of safety than to pressure. When you cultivate predictability, supportive relationships, and regular recovery, stress hormones tend to normalize more quickly after spikes, and the system becomes less jumpy. When we ignore these basics, we often pay for it: rising burnout, sleep problems, and stress-linked conditions even in the young. These issues have many causes, and they are not moral failures; they are signals that our collective rhythms are out of balance.

This is why we must understand Survival and Growth more deeply. In the coming chapters, we'll explore how these modes work in everyday life and, most importantly, how to shift your body gently and gradually toward growth when you notice you're stuck in Survival.

We will emphasize small levers with outsized impact breath patterns, light exposure, movement, rest, meaning, and connection applied with patience, flexibility, and respect for your circumstances. We will not promise cures. We will practice skills.

Let this be your turning point: choose relationship over routine, devotion over raw discipline, and alignment over expectation. When discipline begins to feel like home when your practices are integrated with your values and your biology consistency becomes a form of peace. From that peace, genuine growth becomes possible, one reliable day at a time.

When Effort Becomes a Trap

Let me begin with a simple, familiar story. Imagine a house. Not just any house but an old, sturdy home that has stood for years, maybe generations. Its walls were built to last, its foundations set deep in the earth, and its rooms hold the memory of light, laughter, and easy breath. It was designed to live in relationship with the world, windows open to fresh air, doors welcoming sun and movement, a place where warmth and harmony could settle. Then one day a storm arrives not a drizzle, but a violent squall. Thunder cracks; rain hammers the roof; the wind shakes the beams. Fear rises in the occupants. Instinctively, they act: they bolt the doors, slam the windows, nail boards over every opening, and seal the house against the outside. For a moment, it feels wise. Protective. The house holds; the storm passes; nothing breaks.

But something else happens. The danger moves on, and the boards stay up. Days become weeks, weeks become months. The doors remain locked; the windows stay shut. What felt like safety begins to feel like suffocation. Air that once moved freely grows stale; light that once danced across the floor is lost; silence thickens. Slowly, small failures appear. Mold grows in corners. Dust accumulates on every surface. Pipes corrode without flow. Wires fray. Ventilation clogs. Things start to fail not because the house is weak, but because it was never meant to live in permanent lockdown. Its systems were designed to function with air, light, and exchange. Cut off from those conditions, it declines.

This is what Survival Mode often feels like inside a human body. You encounter a storm of grief, conflict, trauma, rejection, chronic stress and your biology responds as it evolved to do. The nervous system "boards up" to protect you. Muscles tighten, breathing shortens, perception narrows, emotions feel urgent. For a time, this response can be protective. But the risk is not the storm itself; it is forgetting to open back up once the sky clears. If the body stays sealed, if the breath does not deepen, if the shoulders do not soften, if the mind does not receive signals of safety then the very response that guarded you can begin to trap you. Over time, systems meant for connection, restoration, and growth are starved of the conditions they need, not because you are weak or broken, but because you were never designed to live in an emergency posture indefinitely.

What, then, is "Survival Mode" really? It is not merely a mindset and not simply "having a stressful day." It is a whole-body physiological state orchestrated by the autonomic nervous system (ANS) and the brain–body stress circuitry, most notably the sympathetic branch and the hypothalamic–pituitary–adrenal (HPA) axis. When the brain perceives a threat physical, social, or even imagined it rapidly mobilizes. Sympathetic activity rises ("fight-or-flight"), releasing catecholamines such as adrenaline and noradrenaline; the HPA axis increases cortisol. These shifts redirect energy toward immediate coping: heart rate and blood pressure increase; pupils dilate; glucose becomes more available to muscles; attention locks onto potential danger. In parallel, processes that are not essential to immediate survival tend to be dialed down: digestion can slow or become irregular, reproductive investment is deprioritized, tissue repair and some aspects of immunity may be modulated. The exact pattern varies by person and context; some people experience slowed gut motility and constipation, others get urgency and diarrhea; some lose appetite, others feel driven to eat energy-dense foods. The theme is conservation and reprioritization, not moral failure.

Crucially, the brain does not always distinguish perfectly between "objective" danger and "perceived" or symbolic threat. It works on prediction and pattern recognition. A harsh email, a strained conversation, financial uncertainty, social exclusion, or perfectionistic self-criticism can, for many people, trigger physiological responses that resemble those evoked by overt hazards. Modern stressors rarely arrive as a single acute event; they recur, accumulate, and remain unresolved. When stressors become frequent and recovery insufficient, the body's stress systems may spend more time "on" than they were designed to for what researchers sometimes call increased allostatic load. In this state, the system is still trying to help you survive; it simply does so at a cost to long-term balance.

This is why rushing all day without pauses, skipping meals because you're "too busy," chronic multitasking in noisy environments, relentless self-critique, or never allowing rest can keep the nervous system biased toward hyper-vigilance. The ANS is not “logical” in the way a spreadsheet is logical; it is adaptive. It cares less about whether a threat is reasonable than whether patterns have signaled “not safe.” A job rejection is not exile from an ancient tribe, yet the body can react as if exclusion has occurred. Financial worry is not famine, but uncertainty about resources can recruit metabolic and behavioral strategies shaped for scarcity. Conflict with a partner is not an attack by a predator, yet it can activate circuitry calibrated for immediate self-protection. When the “volume” of stress stays high, the emergency settings remain engaged more often, and the long-arc processes of restoration have less room to operate.

Physiologically, that can look like an elevation in baseline arousal, shallower breathing, a quicker heart, sleep that feels light or fragmented, and digestion that is either sluggish or erratic. Hormonal rhythms may shift: cortisol’s daily pattern can flatten or spike at unhelpful times; thyroid and reproductive axes can show downstream effects; immune signaling may tilt toward more inflammatory tone in some people and immunosuppression in others. None of these changes guarantee a specific outcome human bodies are diverse and resilient but they help explain why some people notice bloating or reflux, why others see irregular cycles, why hair shedding can increase (a phenomenon called telogen effluvium during periods of strain), why focus becomes jumpy, or why energy feels thin despite effortful self-care. It is not that healthy actions “don’t count.” It is that the body may be interpreting those actions through the lens of threat rather than safety, and thus allocating resources differently than you intend.

Consider Arjun. On paper, he looks like discipline made human: up at 5:00 a.m., a precise yoga sequence, a 6K run with every split tracked, a cold shower, a carefully measured protein shake and green smoothie, breakfast weighed and logged, journaling, goals, visualizations, affirmations. The schedule is immaculate. But inside, he wakes to tightness, not ease. The first sensation is not gratitude; it is urgency: get up or fall behind. He eats cleanly and yet eats with tension each bite accompanied by a mental audit. If he deviates from the plan, guilt and compensatory strategies flood in. Food becomes a negotiation with fear rather than a conversation with hunger and satiety. At work, he executes flawlessly but from pressure more than purpose; every "send" carries a hum of dread about mistakes, every accomplishment evaporates into the next demand. His calendar leaves no room for softness. Invitations are declined; stillness feels unsafe. Rest is earned, not allowed. Even at bedtime, he aims for 10:30 p.m. because he values recovery, yet his mind continues to sprint, looping through "Did I do enough? What if I slip?" Sleep arrives, but restoration does not always follow; he wakes with the same urgency. Outside, he appears lean, productive, and composed. Inside, he is breathing through a straw.

What's happening for Arjun is not uncommon. His habits are not "bad." Many are health-promoting in the right context. But his nervous system is running them under a chronic threat setting. Motivation science calls this controlled motivation behavior driven by pressure, fear, or guilt versus autonomous motivation behavior aligned with values and a sense of choice. The first can produce compliance; the second is more likely to yield well-being and sustainment. When routines are executed with clenched jaws, the body tends to register the routine as another demand, not a cue of safety. Yes, short-term results can appear: weight can change, fitness can improve, biomarkers can move. But sustainability often hinges on whether the system regularly receives signals that it can downshift and repair. Without those signals, gains may be fragile, and setbacks can feel disproportionate because the body never learned to feel safe in the new patterns.

This is the paradox at the heart of so much modern "discipline." Behaviors that look healthy can be run on a stress engine. Structured meals can signal scarcity if the dominant feeling is "don't mess up." Training can signal an emergency if the story underneath is "outrun failure." Even sleep, the most potent recovery tool we have can be undermined by hyperarousal if the mind treats the night as yet another performance. The result is a life that looks like thriving but feels like surviving. It is not moral weakness; it is a mismatch of inputs: effort without safety, structure without softness, action without recovery.

We have also been sold a narrow story about health: push harder, control more variables, remove more foods, track more metrics, tolerate more discomfort, and you will be well. There is truth here consistency matters; load creates adaptation; inputs shape outcomes. But there is an unpriced cost when effort becomes the only instrument we know how to play. Obsession is not the same as commitment, and guilt is not the same as discipline. A missed workout is often just a data point, not a diagnosis. When the pursuit itself compresses your breath and tightens your chest, the signal may be less about your willpower and more about your physiology asking for conditions it can grow under.

This is not an argument against ambition or structure. It is an invitation to ask a prior question: are our efforts being metabolized as support or as stress? Because in biology, context is often the difference between medicine and burden. Eating nutrient-dense food while feeling safe, connected, and unhurried tends to support digestion and hormonal balance more readily than the same plate eaten under fear. Movement performed with adequate recovery and an internal "yes" is more likely to produce robust, durable adaptations than the same workload performed against a backdrop of threat. Sleep taken in a body that feels protected because the day included moments of downshift does a different kind of work than sleep used only to recharge for another day of battle.

None of this means that people who avoid exercise, eat ultra-processed foods all day, chronically under sleep, or rely on stimulants and late nights are "doing it right." That path also carries risks metabolic, cardiovascular, cognitive, emotional. What this chapter is pointing to is the wide middle: the people striving earnestly, showing up early, eating carefully, training regularly, following plans and yet feeling stuck, inflamed, or exhausted. They have upgraded behaviors but not always the underlying state. Survival Mode has simply been refitted with better habits. The body is still scanning, bracing, and budgeting as though danger is close.

When the nervous system remains chronically tilted toward threat, growth is not impossible, but it is constrained and more costly. Energy is preferentially routed to "now" at the expense of "later." That can look like weight loss that reverses when rigidity eases, blood sugar that improves for a season and then destabilizes under life changes, inflammation that calms but flares with minor disruptions, training progress that plateaus despite effort. These patterns do not mean you failed or lacked willpower. They more often mean the system did not receive enough signals of safety to consolidate the gains. Brains learn through repetition, and bodies adapt through cycles of stress and recovery. If the "stress" portion is ever-present and the "recovery" portion is too brief or tense, the lesson the body encodes is endurance, not ease.

It helps to name the other pole of this continuum what we might call "Growth Mode." This is not a separate on/off switch in the nervous system so much as a shorthand for conditions that support restoration and adaptation: parasympathetic tone that can rise when needed, flexible heart-rate variability, predictable sleep–wake rhythms, nourishment taken with presence, relationships that convey safety, training dosed with recovery, and moments of genuine enjoyment. In Growth Mode, your physiology still responds to challenges, you lift heavy, you sprint, you solve problems but it also receives reliable cues that the challenge is bounded and that repair will happen. Over time, this pattern tends to make change feel more sustainable. It does not guarantee a specific outcome; it creates a climate where outcomes can take root.

So how do we recognize when effort has become a trap? One clue is how your routines feel in your body. If a "healthy" behavior consistently tightens your throat, compresses your breath, or fills your mind with threat-colored thoughts, your nervous system may be interpreting it as pressure. Another clue is your recovery: do you wake restored, or merely reset to "do it again"? Do you have space for spontaneity without fear that everything will unravel? Do you experience moments of softness, pleasure, or unstructured play and can you stay with them without bargaining? None of these pass–fail tests; they are signposts pointing to the state under the strategy.

The aim is not reckless living on one side or rigid living on the other. It is a living posture where discipline is emotionally rooted anchored to values and meaning so that your actions feel like support rather than self-defense. In this posture, eating well often feels like care, not control. Movement feels like strength and presence, not punishment. Rest feels like participation in health, not an indulgence that needs to be justified. You still train hard, but you also downshift; you still track data, but you hold it lightly; you still plan, but you leave room for life.

If you recognize yourself in Arjun, it does not mean you are weak or broken. It means your strategy has been doing the job it was designed to do to keep you going in an environment that rarely signals "safe." The work ahead is not to abandon effort but to rebalance it: to pair your structure with cues of safety, to reintroduce air and light where boards have stayed up too long, to let your system learn that growth is allowed. Changing the state that underlies the strategy will not promise instant transformation, but it can make the changes you earn more likely to last because your body will be able to keep them.

Health should not feel like anxiety wrapped in good intentions. You should be able to eat in peace. You should be able to move for joy and strength. You should be able to rest without guilt, to slow down without fear, and to live in your body without constant bracing. As earlier chapters explored, discipline becomes sustainable when it is connected to why when it is guided by clarity rather than driven by panic. The practical question, then, is how to begin from a state that favors growth rather than survival. How to train, nourish, and recover in ways your biology can register as supportive.

The Healing Loop — How We Shift from Survival to Growth

Let's return to the house. The storm is long gone now. The skies have cleared, the thunder has faded into quiet, and the wind has settled into a soft breeze. Outside, trees stand tall again, birds stitch the morning with song, and the sun lays patient light across the earth. Inside, though, time has stalled. The windows remain latched from within, the doors stay bolted, and heavy curtains keep out the day. What was once a bright, breathing home alive with laughter, airflow, and warmth now sits dim and hushed, a little colder and more fragile with each passing day. It didn't begin as a mistake. Closing it up made sense when danger was real. Boarding the windows and sealing the doors felt like wisdom because, in that moment, it was. Protection is not the enemy. The trouble is that no one returned to tell the house the storm had passed. With every day of stillness, the air thickens; dust gathers; faint threads of mold appear in the undisturbed corners; plumbing dries and stutters; wiring loses resilience; ventilation falters. None of this happens because the house is flawed. It happens because the house was built for exchange of light, movement, connection and the flow was cut off.

Then something shifts, almost too quietly to notice at first. Someone steps back inside not with urgency or a fistful of tools, but with presence. They do not rush. They look around, breathe, and listen to the creaks of the floorboards. They cross the room and ease a window open, just a little enough for a ribbon of air to slip through and for a band of sunlight to reach across the floorboards. They unfasten the door not wide, simply enough for circulation to begin. One board comes down, then another. There is no tearing. There is a release. Dust is lifted, corners are cleared, the small green insistence of life returns in a vase on the table. Music, warm water, laughter signals of safety. The house exhales. The air feels lighter. The systems inside, frozen long enough to feel permanent, begin to stir. Not perfect. Not polished. But open, functional, and safe enough to welcome life back in.

This is what Growth Mode can feel like in a body. It is not a push. It is not a performance. It does not ask you to sprint toward perfection. It is the steady return of flow breath deepening, warmth gathering in the center, lightness in the chest. It looks like the nervous system lowering its guard and tissues softening their brace. It sounds like a quiet message spreading through your internal network: “There is room to recover.” Growth Mode does not mean everything is fixed; it means the constant bracing has eased enough that repair is now possible. From that one shift sometimes subtle, sometimes unmistakable, the work of restoration can begin.

Growth Mode isn't just about feeling good; it's a set of physiological conditions that make healing and adaptation more likely. In scientific terms, it reflects a body spending more time in regulated states: the autonomic nervous system (ANS) shows healthier flexibility; the stress response still rises to meet real demands but returns to baseline more efficiently; and long-arc processes like digestion, tissue repair, immune regulation, and learning gets more reliable access to resources. The essential signal is "safe enough." The brain tracks that perception through interoception (how it senses the body), and those signals shape downstream biology.

Two pathways are especially relevant. First, the ANS balances its sympathetic ("fight or flight") survival mode, and parasympathetic ("rest and repair") growth mode, branches more fluidly. The parasympathetic system communicates heavily through the vagus nerve, a bidirectional highway between body and brain. Slow, diaphragmatic breathing can influence vagal afferents and the baroreflex mechanisms that help smooth heart rhythms and blood pressure changes supporting a calmer baseline. Second, the hypothalamic–pituitary–adrenal (HPA) axis, the hormonal arm of the stress response can show a steadier daily rhythm, with cortisol more aligned to daytime activity and nighttime recovery. These shifts are tendencies rather than guarantees and vary by person and context, but together they create a climate more favorable to repair.

As breathing slows and deepens, gas exchange steadies; oxygen delivery and carbon dioxide clearance adjust in ways the brainstem tracks closely. Circulation redistributes as the body requires less "ready-to-sprint" blood flow to the limbs and can reliably support core functions. In a chronically threatened state, digestion often becomes irregular because the body prioritizes short-term survival. In a more regulated state, the gut tends to re-engage its sequence: salivary enzymes begin the process; gastric acid and pancreatic enzymes are released in better timing; bile flows when needed; and peristalsis the gut's wave-like movement finds a steadier cadence. Many people experience this as less discomfort and more predictable bowel habits, although responses vary and underlying conditions matter. Improving gut function also supports the gut–brain axis, a dense conversation of neural, endocrine, and immune signals that can influence mood, attention, and stress reactivity.

Hormonal systems can settle when the body feels safer. The HPA axis may reduce unnecessary "background" activation, which in turn can support steadier glucose regulation and energy across the day. Thyroid signaling (involving TSH, T4, and T3) is sensitive to illness, inflammation, calorie availability, and stress; when those pressures ease, some people notice a shift toward better subjective energy and temperature comfort, provided their thyroid biology is intact and medical issues are addressed. Sex hormones like estrogen, progesterone, and testosterone respond to sleep, nutrition, activity, and stress exposure; with supportive inputs, cycles can become more predictable and libido and mood may feel more stable. These are patterns, not promises: age, genetics, medications, and health conditions play substantial roles.

Muscles tell the story at the surface. Under pressure, bodies often hold themselves tighter: jaw clenched, shoulders lifted, breath shallow, pelvis braced. In a more regulated state, baseline tone can drop toward a healthier resting set point. Perceived stiffness often eases, range of motion improves, and movement feels less like friction and more like language the body already knows. Because physical training is, by definition, a dose of stress, pairing it with strong recovery signals allows the same workload to produce better adaptations. Sleep is where much of that repair is consolidated. When arousal is lower and circadian cues are honored, light exposure in the morning, dimmer light at night, and consistent timing the brain is more likely to cycle through deeper non-REM stages and REM without frequent awakenings. During these stages, memories are organized; emotional charge can soften; tissues receive growth and repair signals; and brain "housekeeping" processes (studied as the glymphatic system, especially in animal models) appear more active. The outcome, when it happens, is not simply more hours slept but a greater sense of restoration on waking.

Cognition and mood shift alongside the body. As physiology steadies, the prefrontal cortex, the hub for planning, attention, and emotion regulation often has an easier time coordinating with limbic circuits that generate threat responses. People may notice fewer spirals of catastrophic thinking and more room for curiosity and creativity. Emotional reactivity doesn't vanish, but it can become easier to notice early and navigate more skillfully. The broader pattern is a move from reactivity (automatic responses to perceived threat) toward responsiveness (flexible choices attuned to the real situation).

A helpful point often surprises people: long stretches in Growth Mode are not necessary to see benefits. Consistent brief windows even on the order of 10 to 60 minutes across a day can help the nervous system relearn balance. These windows can look modest from the outside: a few minutes of slow nasal breathing; a phone-free walk; a meal eaten without hurry; lying down with eyes closed; or simply pausing to check in with your body before switching tasks. Such practices are not "doing nothing." Biologically, they deliver believable cues of safety. Over time, those cues can accumulate into meaningful change. No single practice guarantees a specific result, but together they shift the background conditions so recovery becomes more available.

Healing rarely emerges from punishment or pressure. It emerges from conditions that permit recovery. When the body senses "safe enough," even briefly, it begins to reopen. Tissues release some grip. Organs recalibrate. The mind is less compelled to brace against imagined futures. In those spaces, energy can return; clarity can flicker back on; immune signaling may quiet from constant high alert; and the background noise of inflammation may ease. Timelines vary. Not every change will be obvious from the outside. But these are the kinds of shifts that allow restoration to take root because the system is no longer spending all of its budget on defense. It lets in the light again.

The Science of the Shift

Your body is not just a collection of organs. It is a living, networked ecosystem made up of interdependent systems: nervous, respiratory, circulatory, muscular, skeletal, digestive, endocrine, immune, urinary, lymphatic, integumentary, reproductive that rarely act alone. In lived physiology they overlap and co-author one another's work. When one part is strained, it tugs the rest. The good news is that interconnection runs both ways. Support a strategically chosen system in a gentle, sensible order and the benefits can ripple outward. That is the heart of the Growth Mode Healing Loop: rather than demanding everything change at once, you apply small, evidence-aligned practices where the body is most ready to say "yes." The first nudge creates momentum. Like a line of dominos, one shift makes the next more likely not by force, but by restoring the conditions under which biology does what it is built to do.

1. **Respiratory System:** We begin with breath not because it's trendy, but because it is both automatic and voluntary, giving you direct access to regulation. Slow, diaphragmatic breathing especially with slightly longer exhales can influence vagal pathways and the baroreflex, nudging autonomic balance toward parasympathetic influence. People often feel this as a tangible softening shoulders drop, the jaw unhooks, attention widens. Breathing well also steadies gas exchange; more predictable carbon

dioxide levels can help stabilize the drive to breathe and reduce sensations of air hunger in some people. Supports: Nervous System

2. **Nervous System:** As breath steadies, the ANS your body's communication backbone often follows. It coordinates muscle tone, heart rhythms, gut motility, and more. The polyvagal framework (an influential, actively studied model) proposes distinct vagal states linked to cues of safety and threat. Its practical wisdom is simple: when the body perceives connection and calm, the repertoire of adaptive responses expands. With more regulated ANS activity, downstream systems have an easier job. Supports: Circulatory System

3. **Circulatory System:** A calmer autonomic tone allows the cardiovascular system to work with less strain. Heart-rate variability can become a more flexible indicator (not a guarantee) of adaptable regulation. Blood flow distributes more evenly, improving oxygen and nutrient delivery while clearing metabolic by-products more efficiently. These changes set the stage for tissues to repair and for movement to feel more available. Supports: Muscular System

4. **Muscular System:** Chronic stress often shows up as subtle bracing, an always-ready stance that consumes energy and amplifies discomfort. As threat tones down, resting muscle tone can ease. Movement begins to feel less like friction and more like a native language. Because training is a

productive stressor, pairing it with recovery adequate fueling, sleep, and downshifted states tends to yield more durable adaptations. Supports: Skeletal System

5. **Skeletal System:** Reduced bracing improves posture and joint loading; aches tied to sustained tension may ease. Bone is dynamic tissue that responds to load, nutrients, and hormones. A well-regulated system tends to deliver these inputs more coherently, supporting alignment and balance and reducing strain on the spine and organs. Supports: Digestive System

6. **Digestive System:** In threat-biased states, digestion often becomes irregular because the body prioritizes immediate survival. As posture opens and systemic tension drops, digestive function generally has an easier time. Blood returns to the gut; the enteric nervous system coordinates motility more effectively; enzymes and bile are secreted with better timing; and nutrient absorption can improve. Calm, unhurried meals often correlate with fewer symptoms, though gastrointestinal diseases and specific intolerances require targeted care. Supports: Endocrine System

7. **Endocrine System:** This is your hormonal fine-tuning network, shaping metabolism, sleep–wake patterns, growth and repair, and reproduction. As digestion stabilizes and stress load decreases, cortisol's daily curve may resemble a gentler wave (higher in the morning, lower in the evening).

Insulin dynamics can smooth with regular meals, consistent movement, and adequate sleep. Thyroid signaling may benefit indirectly as the body stops interpreting everyday life as a crisis. Sex hormones (estrogen, progesterone, testosterone) are highly sensitive to sleep, nutrition, training load, and stress; with supportive inputs, cycles often feel more predictable and mood steadier, always acknowledging individual variability. Supports: Immune System

8. **Immune System:** A substantial proportion of immune activity interfaces with the gut (via gut-associated lymphoid tissue), constantly sampling and learning from what the body encounters. Under chronic stress, immune responses can tilt toward overactivation or sluggishness; in better-regulated states, immune surveillance and inflammatory signaling often look more measured. Practically, some people notice fewer minor infections, quicker recovery, or calmer skin and joints; experiences vary widely. Supports: Urinary System

9. **Urinary System:** With inflammation better managed and cellular by-products handled efficiently, the kidneys can do their precision work filtering blood, excreting wastes like urea and creatinine, and finely regulating electrolytes and acid–base balance. When hydration, nutrition, hormones, and sleep are steadier, fluid regulation often feels more predictable; day-to-day swings in water retention can lessen, though cycles, salt intake,

medications, heat, and other factors remain important. Supports: Lymphatic System

10. **Lymphatic System:** This drainage and immune-transport network benefits from movement and breath. Lymph moves as muscles contract, arteries pulse, and the diaphragm descends, one reason walking and deep breathing can feel clarifying. When lymph flows, tissues feel less congested and immune cells travel more freely to where they are needed. Supports: Integumentary System

11. **Integumentary System (Skin, Hair, Nails):** The outer body often reflects internal trend lines. Clearer skin, stronger nails, and steadier hair shedding can accompany calmer hormones, consistent nutrition, and better sleep, although genetics, age, and dermatologic conditions remain significant determinants. These changes are not merely cosmetic; they can signal improved internal balance. Supports: Reproductive System

12. **Reproductive System:** Highly sensitive to perceived safety, this system often downshifts under sustained stress and re-engages when resources feel reliable. With sustained signals of predictability, cycles may normalize, libido can return, and fertility may be supported always within the limits set by age and health.

Feeds back into: Respiratory System

When reproductive signals stabilize, they can influence breathing patterns' progesterone, for example, increases ventilatory drive in the luteal phase and during pregnancy subtly shifting respiratory tone. In that way, the loop closes back on breath, reminding us that change in one domain is never isolated. The network keeps learning. Progress in real bodies is rarely linear; it is cyclical. You will feel weeks of momentum and, at times, plateaus or backtracks when life is heavy. The aim is not to force a straight line. It is to keep recreating conditions that make restoration possible.

This isn't about fixing everything perfectly or mastering every system before moving forward. It's about creating small, intentional shifts that cascade. The loop mirrors how the body organizes itself. Some systems breathing and autonomic regulation in particular serve as "master regulators," shaping the context in which other processes operate. Starting with them delivers persuasive, low-friction signals that the environment is safe enough to shift from defending to restoring.

From a neuroscience perspective, the loop aligns with interoception and predictive processing: the brain continually forecasts "what state am I in?" and updates those forecasts based on incoming evidence. When your actions supply repeated signals of safety, slow breathing, unhurried meals, restorative sleep, supportive movement the brain updates its model, and physiology follows. The polyvagal framework adds a practical pointer (while research continues to refine it): cues of safety tend to expand your range of adaptive responses. From systems biology, the reasoning is similar: networks change most efficiently when you influence hubs rather than peripherals. From endocrinology and behavioral science, the pattern repeats: stress hormones modulate insulin sensitivity and sex-hormone signaling; small, consistent behaviors compound through habit formation and identity shifts. None of this guarantees a particular outcome, but it improves the odds that your efforts will be metabolized as support rather than more stress.

The best part is that you don't have to force anything. You don't need punishment or perfection. When the right systems are activated in a sensible order starting with breath, calm, and nourishment the body often remembers its own intelligence. Boards come down. Air moves. Light returns. The house becomes a home again not because you renovated every room overnight, but because you restored the basics that allow every room to function.

From the next chapter onward, we will translate these principles into practice. Not through pressure or guilt, and certainly not through punishment. The path will not ask you to add strain to prove commitment. It will invite you to do less, with more presence and better sequencing. We will restore the body as nature tends to: with rhythm, patience, and trust. The order matters because the body has an order. We will go one system at a time, with small shifts that are reasonable to sustain. Over weeks and months, those shifts stop feeling like tasks and start feeling like you. Breath changes. Sleep deepens. Movement feels like participation instead of penance. Eating becomes a relationship rather than a rulebook. When you stop fighting the body and begin listening to it, the body often meets you there. Growth Mode stops being a place you visit only on breaks or retreats and becomes a tone you can touch most days.

This is your new path and the right pace. It starts not with a leap, but with a window opened an inch. Let's begin.

The Beginning of Restoration

Let's begin at the beginning not just of this journey, but of every moment you've ever lived. Breath arrives before language, before memory, before your first step. Your first inhale signaled your arrival; every breath since has traced the rhythm of your days. You did not have to study it or earn it. Breathing is an elegant reflex gifted by biology, always available, always working in the background, holding steady through laughter and tears, through sleepless nights and quiet mornings. When fear rises, breath often turns quick and shallow. When ease returns, breath lengthens and softens. It has mirrored your inner world more faithfully than any diary, yet most of us seldom notice it. We move through crowded hours on autopilot, our breath shrinking to fit the pace. It gets tight. It hides. It recedes into the background right alongside our awareness of our bodies and needs. But what if breath is not meant to be background? What if it is the ground itself the most reliable place to start when you want to restore?

Before you adjust diet, recalibrate sleep, or fine-tune routines, it helps to begin with the signal your body listens to all day: the pattern of your breathing. Breath interacts with the nervous system through networks that monitor carbon dioxide and acidity in the blood, through pressure sensors in vessels, and through pathways, especially the vagus nerve, that influence heart rate, muscle tone, digestion, and stress responses. A slower, steadier pattern tends to cue calm and presence; a tight, rapid pattern tends to cue vigilance and readiness to act. Breath can't guarantee outcomes or replace medical care, but it reliably participates in how your body decides between spending energy on defense or on repair. You don't have to perfect it. You only need to return to it felt, noticed, and trusted so it can help you shift from bracing to softening.

What, then, is the respiratory system you carry with you? It is your moving bridge with the world: air enters, gases exchange, and chemistry resets with every cycle. Oxygen is not exactly "fuel" fats and carbohydrates supply that but oxygen is the final electron acceptor that lets your cells extract energy efficiently in the mitochondria. Without adequate oxygen delivery, cells struggle to maintain that energy economy. Carbon dioxide, meanwhile, is not merely waste. It buffers the blood's pH, helps hemoglobin release oxygen where it's needed (the Bohr effect), and powerfully guides the brainstem's impulse to breathe. The task of respiration, bringing in oxygen, letting go of carbon dioxide, and keeping pH in a healthy range is continuous and exquisitely regulated.

Air ideally enters through the nose. The nasal passages filter particles, warm and humidify air to protect delicate tissues, and modulate flow. Nasal breathing is also associated with small amounts of nitric oxide from the paranasal sinuses, which may support ventilation–

perfusion matching in the lungs; the effect is subtle but potentially helpful. From the nose, air travels past the pharynx and larynx gatekeepers that direct air toward the lungs and protect the airway during swallowing; the larynx also houses the vocal cords, letting breath carry voice, whisper, laughter, and cry. The trachea conducts air toward the bronchi, which branch into bronchioles that end in millions of alveoli. These tiny, thin-walled sacs press breath and blood close enough for diffusion: oxygen slips into the bloodstream while carbon dioxide moves into the airways to be exhaled. The lungs themselves are elastic but largely passive; they inflate and deflate because muscles around them change pressure. Chief among those muscles is the diaphragm, a dome-shaped sheet at the base of the ribcage. When it contracts, it draws downward, enlarging the chest cavity and gently pulling air in. Intercostal muscles between the ribs assist, fine-tuning the expansion. With each cycle, your body quietly balances chemistry, temperature, and pressure in service of stable internal conditions.

This automatic choreography is guided by centers in the brainstem that integrate signals from chemoreceptors (monitoring CO_2, O_2, and pH) and mechanoreceptors (sensing stretch). Yet breathing is unique among autonomic functions: you can choose to influence it. You cannot decide your blood pressure on command, but you can slow an exhale, soften a breath hold, or return to nasal breathing. When you do, you send measurable ripples through the autonomic nervous system. Slow, comfortable breathing commonly around four to six breaths per minute for many adults, though the ideal pace varies tends to strengthen respiratory sinus arrhythmia, the natural rise and fall of heart rate with breath. That pattern reflects healthy vagal modulation of the heart and is often experienced as settling. Emphasizing an unhurried exhale can enhance this effect for some people, likely by increasing parasympathetic influence and engaging baroreflex pathways that help the heart and blood vessels find a steadier rhythm. None of this is a cure-all, but together it is a practical way to bias the system toward recovery.

Why begin here? Because breath is an accessible lever. When the day accelerates and the mind races, breathing often follows shallow, quick, upper-chest. That pattern is a useful part of the "fight or flight" response when you truly need to mobilize, but if it becomes your baseline, the body may keep acting as if a threat is near. Stress hormones surge more often, digestion takes a back seat, muscles stay primed, and attention narrows. By contrast, when you slow and deepen the breath, especially with a softer, longer exhale, you tilt the physiology away from constant mobilization and toward restoration. Heart rate tends to decrease. Skeletal muscle tone eases. Blood flow redistributes to support digestion. Inflammation-related signals can trend downward over time. Mood and attention can feel more stable. These shifts are averages, not guarantees, but they are consistent enough across studies and experience to make breath a sensible first step.

Beginning does not require ceremony. It requires sincerity. Lie down if you can, on a floor or firm surface, and let gravity do the first work. Unclench the jaw.

Soften the abdomen. Place a hand over the lower ribs or belly to feel movement. Invite the breath through the nose; allow the abdomen to rise as the diaphragm descends, then let the abdomen fall as the exhale arrives on its own. Imagine the inhale like a gentle tide advancing, and the exhale like a tide receding no rush, no force. If it helps, picture the lower ribs expanding in a soft ring, the back of the ribcage widening into the floor, the collarbones staying relatively quiet. If counting supports ease, you might explore a light pattern such as a comfortable inhale and a slightly longer exhale, but let numbers serve you, not rule you. The aim is comfort, not performance.

You may notice yawns. That's common when arousal shifts. Science has not settled on a single explanation for yawning; hypotheses include transitions in vigilance, regulation of brain temperature, and subtle adjustments in pressure and gases. In practice, a yawn during gentle breathing often coincides with muscles letting go and attention widening. You can let it happen without reading too much into it.

As the breath finds a natural rhythm and the sense of effort fades, you may choose to sit. There is no prize for lotus pose. A sturdy chair is perfect. Rest both feet on the ground. Let the spine be long but not rigid, as if a thread lifts the crown of the head while the tailbone drops heavy. Soften the glutes and shoulders. Keep the tongue loose in the mouth and the gaze soft. The instructions remain the same: nasal inhale with the diaphragm leading, unforced exhale that lingers a touch longer. Feel the lower ribs like wings that open and close. Let the breath become quiet enough to be invisible from across the room yet vivid enough to be unmistakable from the inside.

The goal is not to become a specialist in techniques. Advanced pranayama and other breath practices can be profound and, when learned with care, may unlock new capacities. But timing matters. Most bodies benefit first from restoring easy diaphragmatic motion and a relaxed cadence before layer-ing in holds, ratios, or forceful patterns. Think of it like strength training: you establish range and control with light load before attempting heavy lifts. If breath tightens, if the throat catches or the shoulders hike, that is useful data. Back off. Return to comfort. Let ease be the metric.

You don't need dedicated blocks of time to benefit. Micro-pauses scattered through the day are remarkably potent. Before you open your laptop, take two slow nasal breaths. After a difficult message, take three. Lying in bed upon waking, follow five gentle cycles and feel the abdomen rise and fall under your palm. Standing in a queue, rest your attention on the breath rather than on the nearest screen. Before you eat, take a few unhurried exhales to cue "rest and digest." These moments won't erase stressors, but they can help your physiology visit calmer states more often, and the nervous system learns from repetition.

This is a quiet form of rebellion in a culture that celebrates constant acceleration. It doesn't announce itself. It does not demand the perfect mat or room or schedule. It asks only for presence. When you reclaim your breath, you are not just moving air; you are participating in how your body allocates its energy less toward bracing, more toward repair. Muscles that have been holding on may release a little. The jaw can unclench. The heart, used to rushing, may find a steadier rhythm. The mind, always scanning for what's next, can receive a credible message from within: for this moment, you are safe enough to soften.

None of this overrides the value of medical assessment and care. If you live with respiratory, cardiovascular, neurological, or mental-health conditions or if breathing practices make you dizzy, short of breath, or uncomfortable consult a qualified professional and adapt as needed. Breathing practices are supportive tools, not replacements for treatment.

As breath begins to move more freely, you may notice something else: other systems start to cooperate. The digestive tract, richly innervated and exquisitely sensitive to stress, often functions more comfortably when the autonomic pendulum swings toward rest. The immune system, which communicates closely with stress pathways, may shift away from constant red alert when the body perceives less threat. Hormones involved in energy, appetite, and sleep can find steadier patterns when the nervous system is not constantly being asked to sprint. These are tendencies, not promises, but they are the kinds of shifts that accumulate.

Every breath is a small conversation with your body. With a hurried inhale and clipped exhale, the message sounds like "get ready." With a smooth, deep inhale and a longer, softer exhale, the message sounds more like "you can release." Restoration rarely arrives through force. It arrives through rhythm through signals repeated gently, often, and credibly enough that the body believes them. You do not need to wait for the perfect window. You do not need to perform. You only need to pause and participate.

This is why the respiratory system is the first door we open. It is not just a set of tubes and sacs; it is a signaling network woven into every other system you depend on. Inhale. Exhale. Again. With each cycle, you are teaching your physiology at a different pace. You are building a bridge from the outside world to the inside, from noise to nuance, from bracing to trust.

And as that bridge strengthens, the next chapter comes into clearer view. The nervous system, the command center that records experience and shapes habits of protection listens closely to breath. It is sculpted by what has happened to you and how your body learned to stay safe. In the pages ahead, we'll explore how those patterns form and how, with the steady guidance of breathing and other gentle practices, you can lead the system back toward clarity and ease. For now, keep it simple. Let the breath be felt, not forced. Let it carry you at your pace, in your way. This is not just breathing. This is the beginning of restoration.

From Defense to Restoration

Let's begin with a quiet truth that shapes every corner of health: when your biology leans hard toward protection, most other priorities are throttled down. You can eat well, train consistently, and take thoughtful supplements, yet if your body keeps receiving "danger" signals, it will continue to allocate energy toward short-term safety rather than long-term repair. Digestion may slow, sleep may feel light or broken, the immune response may become harder to regulate, and hormones that steer energy and mood can drift from their usual patterns. None of this means you are weak or faulty; it means your body is following instructions. And the primary source of those instructions is the system that decides how vigilant or how restful you'll be, is your nervous system.

Though it is not visible like muscle or skin, the nervous system is the most pervasive messenger you have. It is the coordination hub that links brain, spinal cord, and the farthest cells at your fingertips and toes, conducting a ceaseless flow of electrical impulses and chemical signals. Through it you sense heat and pressure, move a limb, form a memory, react to a surprise, and recover after effort. Beyond these obvious functions, it also shapes your internal landscape: how safe you feel, how quickly you calm after stress, how efficiently your gut moves food forward, how readily you fall asleep, and how much energy is available for the quiet work of maintenance. When stressors arrive whether an actual threat or a thought that the brain interprets as one this same system can shift the whole body toward a defensive stance. In that stance, healing is not impossible, but it is harder; the organism prioritizes "handle this now" over "repair for later."

At a structural level, the nervous system has two broad divisions. The central nervous system (CNS) brain and spinal cord, is the processing center, integrating input and sending out commands. The peripheral nervous system (PNS) carries those commands and returns information from skin, muscles, joints, and organs. Within the PNS there are two major functional streams. The somatic branch governs voluntary movement and sensory input you're aware of picking up a cup, feeling the texture of cloth. The autonomic nervous system (ANS) regulates functions you do not usually control directly: heart rhythm, blood vessel tone, sweat, gut motility and secretions, aspects of immune–inflammatory responses, and elements of temperature regulation. Many researchers also treat the enteric nervous system, the dense nerve network of the gastrointestinal tract as a semi-independent partner that communicates constantly with both brain and immune cells.

The ANS is often described as having two complementary arms. The sympathetic branch primes the body for action: it can accelerate heart rate, redirect blood flow toward skeletal muscle, dilate pupils, and mobilize stored energy. This "fight-or-flight" pattern is adaptive and lifesaving when fast responses are needed. The parasympathetic branch, strongly mediated by the vagus nerve among others, supports "rest-and-digest" activities: it can help slow heart rate, promote gut motility and secretions, and bias the body toward repair and immune surveillance. In daily life, these branches are not literal on/off switches; they often co-activate in nuanced ways, blending to meet the moment. Too much sympathetic drive for too long can feel like chronic tension or hypervigilance; too little can feel flat or sluggish. Health is less about silencing one branch and more about flexible regulation mounting an appropriate response when needed and returning, reliably, to baseline.

Modern life is rich in cues that the body may interpret as "handle this now": deadlines, notifications, conflict, noise, uncertainty, even harsh self-talk. None of these are predators, yet many of them recruit similar circuitry. Over time, repeated activation can produce allostatic load, the wear and tear that accumulates when systems designed for short bursts of stress are engaged too frequently or for too long. Allostatic load does not break you; it strains capacity. Digestion may become sensitive, sleep may become lighter, inflammatory signaling may be harder to settle, and attention may narrow. Naming this pattern is not to dramatize it but to make sense of it: your body is working hard to keep you safe with the information it is receiving.

This is why the nervous system sits so close to the center of any healing sequence. It is both historian and gatekeeper. It records experience not only as facts or images but as patterns in muscle tone, heart rhythm, breathing, and hormonal cascades. Protective strategies can become familiar enough that calm feels foreign and vigilance feels normal. None of this is a personal failing. It is plasticity, the nervous system learning what it needs to learn to carry you through. The work ahead is not forceful "fixing." It is creating conditions in which the system can update its priors and discover, by experience, that it is allowed to downshift.

Breath is a practical place to begin making those conditions as you explored in the previous chapter because respiration is both automatic and voluntary. Rhythm generators in the brainstem keep you breathing without effort, while the cortex can adjust rate and depth. Slow, comfortable breathing, especially with a slightly longer exhale, tends to enhance vagal modulation of the heart (often felt as steadier, calmer beats) and to nudge baroreflexes and other feedback loops toward balance. Breath is not a magic key, but it is a credible, repeatable signal. Once that signal is established, attention can widen to the broader nervous system, the set of pathways that must interpret the invitation and allow the body to accept it.

To understand how this acceptance unfolds, it helps to look briefly at the chemistry of stress and ease. During threat, the sympatho-adrenal system releases catecholamines such as adrenaline and noradrenaline, and the hypothalamic-pituitary-adrenal (HPA) axis increases cortisol. Acutely, these are helpful: they sharpen focus, mobilize fuel, and suppress functions not immediately required for escape. With time and repetition, though, the baseline of these signals can drift; sleep architecture can shift toward lighter, more fragmented patterns; the gut's rhythm and sensitivity can change; and immune messaging can oscillate in ways that make inflammation more likely to flare or linger. Conversely, cues of safety: social connection, predictable routines, unhurried breathing, a sense of agency tend to rebalance these networks. None of this guarantees specific clinical outcomes, but these trends are well described across physiology and psychology: the more often the body visits regulated states, the easier it becomes to return to them.

Restoring the nervous system, then, is not a single technique but a family of gentle inputs that add up. Mindfulness practices are among the best studied. In particular, body-scan meditation systematically placing attention on one region of the body at a time appears to strengthen interoception (the sense of internal signals) and to engage brain regions involved in monitoring and regulation. Neuroimaging studies often implicate the insula and anterior cingulate cortex in these shifts, though findings vary by method and population. What matters for practice is simple: repeatedly noticing sensations without judgment teaches the system that you will listen. That listening reduces the need for the body to shout via tension or pain.

A body scan does not require silence or a special room. You can lie on a mat, sit in a supportive chair, or rest in bed. Close the eyes if comfortable, soften the jaw and belly, and begin with the smallest places perhaps the toes. Attend to temperature, pressure, tingling, or the absence of sensation. After a few breaths, move gradually to the soles, ankles, calves, knees, and so on, traveling up through hips and abdomen, ribcage and back, shoulders and arms, neck, scalp, and face. If you notice areas that feel tight, simply acknowledge them; if an area feels blank or distant, that too is information. Let the breath wander in the background without forcing it. When you reach the end, widen your attention to include the whole body at once, as if you were listening to a chorus rather than a solo. Five minutes is enough to begin. Longer is fine if it remains comfortable. Consistency matters more than duration.

Other practices can complement this foundation. Humming, chanting, or extended "voiced" exhales lengthen the out-breath and add gentle vibration in the throat and chest; whether or not they directly stimulate the vagus nerve, they often make slow breathing easier and more pleasant. Gargling engages cranial nerves in the throat and can be a playful way to cue attention to this area, though direct evidence for strong physiologic effects is limited. Self-massaging your scalp, jaw, neck, forearms, hands, feet can downshift muscle guarding and increase the sense of safety in the skin and fascia (the body reads touch as context). Progressive muscle relaxation alternates deliberate tension and release, helping you feel the difference between bracing and letting go. Mindful walking synchronizes step and breath; even a few laps at home can re-introduce rhythm after screen time. Gentle stretching of large, tolerant muscle groups calves, quadriceps, chest can widen range without provoking the reflex to protect. None of these is required; any of them can help. Choose what your body meets with the least resistance.

As you explore, keep expectations realistic and kind. You are not turning off the sympathetic system (you need it), nor are you chasing a permanent parasympathetic glow (too much can be unhelpful, as anyone who has fainted from a sudden vagal surge knows). You are cultivating flexibility, the capacity to mobilize when appropriate and to settle when the moment has passed. Signs that flexibility is improving tend to be modest and practical: the jaw unclenches more easily after a hard conversation; the stomach handles a meal with less complaint; sleep becomes a little deeper or easier to return to after waking; focus lasts a bit longer before the urge to scroll wins. Over weeks and months, these small changes can cumulate. If practices consistently produce dizziness, distress, or breathlessness or if you live with medical or mental-health conditions, partnering with a qualified clinician can help tailor the work.

The language of safety "you can soften now" is poetic, but it also reflects biology. The nervous system relies on prediction: based on past experience, it estimates what the next moment demands and prepares physiology accordingly. When it regularly receives credible evidence that the current moment is safe enough, friendly faces, tolerable sensations, predictable routines, small successes it recalibrates those predictions. Your digestive tract, richly innervated and closely linked to mood through immune and hormonal messengers, often functions more smoothly when threat levels drop. Sleep architecture often improves as hyperarousal fades. Hormonal axes that govern energy, appetite, and stress can find steadier patterns. None of this occurs overnight or in a straight line, and none of it removes the need for medical care when it is indicated. But the trend is clear: restoration becomes more likely when the organism trusts that it can afford to restore.

This chapter does not ask you to adopt a rigid regimen. It asks for rhythm. Scatter short practices across the day rather than forcing long sessions that you dread. Two unhurried breaths before you open a message. A one-minute scan of jaw, shoulders, and belly between meetings. A slow walk to the sink and back, matching three steps to the inhale and four to the exhale. A warm hand on the sternum as you lie down to sleep. These micro-signals are small, but repetition matters. Biology learns by frequency.

What we're doing here is not "hacking." We are honoring systems that have worked diligently on your behalf through every season, even the hard ones. You are showing your body, again and again, that it does not need to hold its breath around you. The message is simple, delivered in many dialects: breath, touch, movement, attention: you are safe enough, for this moment, to release some of the guard. When that message lands consistently and without pressure patterns begin to shift. Digestion can resume its rhythm. Sleep can deepen. Energy that once fueled constant scanning can be reallocated toward learning, repair, and creation.

The body never intended to live in perpetual emergency; it was waiting for conditions to change.

Those conditions are now taking shape. Through your breathing practice, through a gentle body scan, through small acts of self-care repeated often, you are providing credible evidence of safety. That evidence does not erase old imprints, but it does give the nervous system new material. In time, trust grows not as an abstract ideal, but as a felt sense: muscles no longer braced by default, a heart that settles more quickly, a mind that can widen its view. Trust is not the end of healing; it is the ground on which healing stands.

From here, the next step in the sequence becomes natural. Safety does not only rest; it also moves. Once the nervous system spends more time in regulated states, the circulatory system can be engaged more intentionally not with strain, but with supportive flow. Circulation carries oxygen, nutrients, warmth, and immune cells to where they are needed and clears what is no longer useful. It is one of the ways safety is distributed through the body, turning local ease into whole-body cooperation. That is where we will go next. For now, pause. Let this settling register. You do not need to race ahead. You have already done something meaningful: you have shown your nervous system that it is allowed to stop protecting all the time and start restoring more of the time. That shift, quiet and cumulative changes what becomes possible.

The Transportation Ways

There is something most of us notice only when it falters: flow. We crave energy, chase clarity, and strive for strength, yet the substrate beneath all three is quiet movement not only of limbs in space but of life within you. Vitality is not just muscle or will; it is distribution. And the system that distributes delivering, collecting, signaling, and balancing moment by moment is one of the most extraordinary and under-appreciated networks you carry: the circulatory system. Even on the days you feel stuck, your blood continues its rounds. Even when emotions grow heavy, your heart keeps time. Even when thoughts scatter, your vessels still adjust minute arteries constricting and dilating, capillaries opening and closing so oxygen, nutrients, heat, hormones, and immune cells can reach the places that need them. You may not feel this choreography, but it is constant. Estimates suggest that an adult's blood vessels ranging from large elastic arteries to microscopic capillaries only five to ten micrometers wide span on the order of 60,000 miles (about 100,000 kilometers). This network warms cool hands, feeds a tired brain, flushes the face in laughter, and pales the skin during fear. The thread running through it all is flowing.

When flow is limited, recovery often feels limited. Circulation is not only heart rate and blood pressure, as important as those are. It is delivery and pickup, coordination and conversation. Your breath may be steadier and your nervous system more settled, but if oxygen, glucose, amino acids, electrolytes, hormones, and immune mediators do not reliably reach tissues and if carbon dioxide and metabolic byproducts are not carried away repair slows. Fatigue lingers. Local inflammation can simmer. Cells, which are always doing their best with what arrives, simply do not receive enough of what they need or cannot offload what they are finished with. Before rebuilding strength or asking muscles for power, there is a more foundational step: restore flow. Flow is how healing travels from a signal to a system.

To understand how to restore it, it helps to know what "circulatory system" really means. At its simplest, it is your internal transport and communication network. The heart is the pressure generator, a fist-sized pump beating roughly one hundred thousand times per day at rest, speeding during effort and settling during sleep, responsive to emotion, posture, temperature, and even the phases of your breath. The vessels are the conduits, but they are also intelligent regulators: large elastic arteries absorb and release pressure with each beat, muscular arteries and arterioles tune regional blood flow by constricting or dilating, veins and venules return blood to the heart with the help of one-way valves and the squeezing action of surrounding muscles, and capillaries provide the exchange surface where blood and tissues meet. It is in these thin-walled capillaries that oxygen leaves hemoglobin and dissolves into the interstitial fluid, carbon dioxide and other wastes return to the circulation, and hormones and nutrients pass into the neighborhoods where they are needed. Exchange does not happen directly with the inside of a cell but across the space between vessels and cells; from there, diffusion and transport carry resources inward.

Blood itself is not just "red liquid." It is a dynamic tissue. Plasma, the fluid portion is mostly water (about 90%) with dissolved proteins, electrolytes, lipids, and signaling molecules; whole blood also contains red cells to carry oxygen, white cells to defend and coordinate immune responses, and platelets to support clotting. At rest, the entire blood volume typically completes a circuit of the body on the order of once a minute, faster during exertion and slower in deep rest. In the lungs, inhaled oxygen diffuses into the blood; in the periphery, oxygen diffuses into tissues. Carbon dioxide, produced by metabolism, returns in dissolved form, bound to proteins, or as bicarbonate to be exhaled. The endothelium, the single-cell lining of every vessel, is an active organ, sensing the shear stress of flowing blood and releasing substances such as nitric oxide that relax vessel walls, reduce friction, and help regulate clotting and inflammation. Healthy flow keeps this endothelial conversation constructive; disrupted flow can make it more reactive.

A few clarifications help keep the map accurate. Arteries generally carry blood away from the heart and veins return it, but oxygen content depends on the circuit:

systemic arteries usually carry oxygen-rich blood to the body while pulmonary arteries carry oxygen-poor blood to the lungs; systemic veins return oxygen-poor blood, and pulmonary veins return oxygen-rich blood to the heart. Capillaries are smaller than a human hair by an order of magnitude, and their permeability varies by tissue so each organ gets what it needs with the right degree of selectivity. The circulatory system also works alongside the lymphatic system, which collects excess interstitial fluid, returns it to the bloodstream, and ferries immune cells—another quiet avenue by which "flow" supports healing.

This network is mechanical, chemical, and also responsive to your internal state. The autonomic nervous system continuously adjusts heart rate and vascular tone; stress can nudge blood away from the skin and gut toward skeletal muscle, sharpening readiness at the expense of digestion, temperature comfort, or skin repair. Safety can allow the reverse. These are not moral judgments; they are allocation decisions made quickly and often. Your face flushing during embarrassment or turning pale during fear is not "in your head", it is your vasculature responding to signals.

In the healing sequence you are following, the circulatory system comes third not because it is less important than breath or the nervous system, but because it depends on them. Breath is how oxygen arrives, and the nervous system is how vascular tone is set. When breathing is steadier and the body is spending more time in regulated states, the signal is ready to be distributed. The circulatory system is that distribution. If vessels are chronically constricted in one region or blood moves sluggishly in another, the benefits of quieter breathing and calmer arousal can remain local rather than global. When flow improves, many people notice practical shifts: thinking feels clearer as neurovascular coupling delivers blood where the brain is active; muscles recover more comfortably because nutrients arrive and byproducts leave; gut motility steadies as perfusion and autonomic tone cooperate; skin looks more vibrant as microcirculation improves; effort feels more doable because oxygen transport and extraction are better matched. These changes are tendencies, not guarantees, and they unfold over weeks to months with repetition, but they describe what happens when distribution catches up with intention.

Restoring flow rarely asks for extremes. In bodies that have been living in survival mode, very high intensity can spike stress chemistry and make it harder to sustain a practice. What circulation responds to best is rhythm, regular, manageable inputs that endothelium, heart, and vessels can trust. Hydration is one quiet input. Because plasma is mostly water, adequate fluid supports blood volume and helps keep viscosity from drifting upward. Dehydration raises plasma osmolality and can make the heart work harder to maintain output; over hydration is not the goal either, so “enough” will vary with body size, temperature, activity, and diet. Beginning the day with water, noticing thirst cues, and spacing fluids across waking hours are simple ways to support the river you depend on.

Another input is simply interrupting stillness. Sitting or standing motionless for long stretches allows blood to pool in the legs and can leave the brain feeling foggy. The calf muscles are sometimes called the "peripheral heart" because each contraction squeezes veins and pushes blood uphill through one-way valves. Standing up briefly each hour, rolling the ankles, or performing a comfortable set of heel raises or ankle pumps can refresh venous return and lighten the legs. The same logic applies to the lymphatic system, which relies on bodily movement and pressure changes rather than a central pump; gentle motion helps it carry fluid and immune cells back to the bloodstream.

Gentle, regular aerobic movement is a cornerstone for many people. Moderate-intensity activities such as brisk walking, relaxed cycling, easy swimming, or dancing at a conversational pace create steady shear stress along vessel walls, a stimulus that tends to improve endothelial function and arterial flexibility over time. With weeks to months of consistency, the heart often becomes more efficient, resting heart rate may decrease, and blood pressure can trend toward healthier ranges if it is elevated. New capillaries may sprout in trained muscles, a process sometimes called angiogenesis or vascular remodeling, improving local delivery and waste removal. Mood often benefits as well, through a tapestry of mechanisms that includes autonomic balance, endocannabinoid signaling, and changes in inflammatory mediators. You do not have to carve a single long session out of your day to begin feeling these effects. Two fifteen-minute walks or three ten-minute strolls, particularly after meals, can support blood sugar handling and endothelial health while keeping effort gentle. If joints are sensitive, water-based exercise or a stationary bike can reduce impact while preserving rhythm.

When pain, time demands, or mobility make even short walks difficult, position can become your ally. Elevating the legs while resting them on a chair or sliding them up a wall while you lie on your back uses gravity to assist venous return, can reduce ankle swelling, and often feels soothing. Breathing slowly in this position may further downshift arousal and help the heart settle. Some people also explore gentle, supported inversions from yoga traditions; these can be relaxing, but they are not necessary for healthy circulation and are not appropriate for everyone. Eye conditions like glaucoma, certain hernias, uncontrolled hypertension, pregnancy after the first trimester, and some neck or spine issues are examples where medical guidance matters. If you try any inversion, make it short, comfortable, and fully supported, and discontinue if you feel pressure, dizziness, or strain.

All of these practices interact. Breathing influences the "respiratory pump," the pressure changes in the chest that draw venous blood toward the heart with each inhale and allow it to move forward with each exhale. Posture affects how freely the diaphragm can descend, which in turn affects both breathing and venous return. The nervous system sets baseline vascular tone and heart rhythm, which determine how readily blood redistributes to meet local demand. Movement provides shear stress and the muscular squeeze that keeps fluids from stagnating. Hydration maintains the medium in which all these adjustments occur. None of these inputs needs to be perfect. What matters most is their rhythm and credibility, small, repeatable signals your body can believe.

If you prefer an outline you can feel rather than count, you might imagine your day as a sequence of gentle nudges. After waking, drink water and take a slow minute to breathe. During work, stand or move each hour just enough to ask your calves and hips to join the day. Sometime before dusk, take a moderate walk or cycle at a pace where conversation is easy and breath stays through the nose; if time is tight, split it into shorter bouts. After the evening meal, stroll for ten minutes to help blood and glucose find their way. Before bed, lie down and rest your legs on a cushion or against the wall, letting breath lengthen on the way out. Spread these nudges across the week. They do not have to be large to be effective; they have to be lived often enough that your vessels, heart, and endothelium adapt.

As flow improves, many people notice shifts that are modest at first and meaningful over time. Hands and feet that were often cold feel warmer as small vessels respond more flexibly. Legs feel less heavy at day's end as venous return keeps pace with gravity. Thinking feels clearer when the brain receives blood where and when it is needed, a process called neurovascular coupling. Breathing feels more coordinated with effort. Recovery between tasks shortens. Skin may look more vibrant as microcirculation improves. Digestion can become more comfortable as perfusion and autonomic tone support its rhythm. These are not promises, and they do not replace medical care when it is needed, but they are the kinds of changes that tend to follow when distribution joins regulation.

It is worth naming cautions alongside encouragement. If you live with cardiovascular, metabolic, hematologic, or vascular conditions; if you have symptoms like chest discomfort, unexplained shortness of breath, fainting, new swelling, severe leg pain, or vision changes; or if exercise and positional changes bring on worrisome sensations, partnering with a qualified clinician is wise. The practices in this chapter are designed to be gentle and supportive, yet individual bodies differ, and tailoring is part of care.

Flow is not only physical. It is also the embodied sense that resources can reach where they are needed. When you restore circulation, you are not just moving blood; you are allowing a feeling of "enough" to travel. Oxygen helps the brain think more clearly; nutrients help tissues repair with less argument; immune cells patrol without overreacting; hormones signal with steadier timing. The message carried by each heartbeat, subtle and repeated, is that energy can be allocated to something other than constant defense. That message does not arrive all at once. It arrives as a hundred quiet deliveries each day, none heroic on its own, together amounting to a shift you can live in.

From here, the sequence you have been following begins to touch the body's structure more directly. When flow improves, muscles often respond. They are not only engines of motion; they are also stabilizers, shock absorbers, and, for many of us, places where we have stored bracing. In a world that moves quickly, muscles frequently hold what has gone unprocessed, tension against the next demand, guarding against the next impact. The next chapter turns toward them with the same spirit that has guided you so far: not to force or harden, but to offer softness, stability, and space. You will not be asked to push through pain or chase a performance. You will be invited to feel what is there and to let go of what no longer needs to be held.

For now, allow the simplicity of this moment to matter. Breathe in with enough depth to feel your ribs widen. Breathe out long enough to feel weight return to the chair or floor. Sense the quiet labor of your heart, the sensitivity of your vessels, the subtle warmth that spreads when flow is unimpeded. You are not stuck; you are circulating. And as circulation returns, restoration becomes something your body can distribute not just to one organ or one mood, but across the whole terrain of you. That shift does not solve everything, and it does not need to. It simply changes what is possible, and over time, possibility changes everything.

Movement Is the Message

Let's begin with a truth that sounds simple but is easy to forget in a sitting world: muscles are not decorations; they are instruments of life. They did not evolve for aesthetics or applause. They evolved so you can reach, lift, carry, climb, brace, speak, chew, blink, breathe, tremble when grief arrives, and dance when joy returns. Movement is not an optional extra layered on top of health it is one of health's foundations. Biologically, skeletal muscle is built to respond to use. Ask it to work and it adapts, coordination improves, strength and endurance rise, joints feel better supported. Stop asking and it adapts in the other direction fibers shrink (atrophy), neural drive fades, movement patterns narrow, and other tissues absorb loads they weren't meant to bear. None of this is a moral judgment. It is the body's remarkable responsiveness.

Modern routines often pull us toward stillness. Hours slip by with hips folded and shoulders rounded as attention stays glued to near objects and small gestures. The body, always learning, takes the hint. Muscles lose conditioning; joints feel "stuck" not because their hinges are broken, but because the nervous system has fewer reasons to allow broad ranges; connective tissues remodel to the loads they see and become less springy;

discomfort grows from a whisper to a conversation and sometimes to a shout. Age plays a role in these changes, but inactivity is the stronger author. The good news is the same plasticity that responds to disuse will respond to considerate use. If we want to truly restore the muscular system, not only shape it, but invite it back into partnership, the beginning is not a supplement stack or a spreadsheet. It is movement: daily, rhythmic, intentional, and kind. Movement nourishes muscle, supports circulation, bathes cartilage in synovial fluid, improves oxygen delivery, and reminds the brain that the body is capable. Movement is how the body remembers itself.

The muscular system is more than the big movers we name in the mirror. It is the engine that powers posture and gesture as well as locomotion. Skeletal muscles keep you upright against gravity, stabilize joints so they can travel safely through their arcs, and share impact so cartilage and ligaments are not overrun. During contraction they generate heat, buffering your core temperature. Their rhythmic squeezing helps venous blood return from the legs toward the heart, and their motion encourages lymph, the immune-rich fluid that drains tissues to flow. Even basic breathing relies on muscle: your diaphragm and intercostals are skeletal muscles whose coordinated contractions change chest pressure so air can move; during higher demand, accessory muscles assist. Inside the body, other muscle types carry out essential work you rarely notice. Smooth muscle surrounds hollow organs and blood vessels; it propels food through the digestive tract (peristalsis), regulates blood pressure by changing vessel diameter, and adjusts airflow in the bronchi. Cardiac muscle, unique to the heart, contracts in a steady rhythm generated by specialized pacemaker cells and guided by electrical pathways; beat by beat, it keeps flow moving. These three tissues: skeletal, smooth, and cardiac differ in structure and control, but together they allow you to inhabit and act in the world.

Skeletal muscle deserves special attention here because it is the part you can influence most directly. Each muscle is a bundle of fibers connected to the tendon, which anchors into bone. Nerves branch into the tissue to form motor units (a motor neuron and all the fibers it commands). When you choose to move or when reflexes choose for you, motor units fire in patterns that create force and direction. Early gains in strength come primarily from the nervous system learning to recruit what you already have, to coordinate partners and opponents, and to quiet unhelpful co-contractions. With sustained, appropriate challenge and adequate recovery, fibers themselves remodel: protein synthesis increases, mitochondria become more capable, capillaries proliferate, and the connective scaffolding that transmits force becomes more organized. The same adaptability underlies loss when the signal is "don't use this." Disuse reduces motor drive and fiber size, and it can blur the brain's "map" of a body part until practice redraws it.

This is one reason the muscular system appears fourth in the healing sequence. In bodies living on high alert, muscles often default to guarding: the jaw tenses, shoulders creep upward, hips hold, the low back grips not because heavy loads are present, but because vigilance is. That background contraction compromises coordination and shrinks comfortable ranges, and joints that are "held" rather than moved tend to feel older than they are. Trying to impose intense training on a system still bracing often yields pain, fatigue, or injury. Breath, nervous-system regulation, and restored circulation change the context in which muscles operate. When those conditions improve, muscles are more willing to lengthen when asked, to contract cleanly when needed, and to share load across chains rather than letting one region carry everything.

"Movement is medicine" is a useful phrase if we remember that dosing and context matter. The aim is not maximal strain; it is credible signals, repeated often enough to reshape capacity without provoking defense. Restoration begins with connection. You cannot strengthen a muscle you cannot feel. Mirrors and metrics can help, but attention helps more. Slow a movement and you'll notice which muscles are doing the work and which are avoiding it. As clarity grows, coordination improves, and strength becomes easier, and safer, to add.

Because "move more" is vague, it helps to understand the qualities of movement that, woven together, build resilient musculature. One quality is resistance: asking muscles to produce force against something that pushes back gravity, your bodyweight, a band, a dumbbell. Thoughtful resistance work recruits motor units more fully, teaches cleaner firing patterns, and supports bone and tendon by applying mechanical stress they require to stay strong. Another quality is power: force applied quickly. Power declines faster with age than strength does, yet can be trained with very small, playful bouts once basic control is present: a light step and lift, a soft landing from a tiny hop, a brisk drive up a single stair, a gentle medicine-ball toss. Intent is crispness, not exhaustion. A third quality is endurance: time under manageable load. Longer walks, easy circuits, stair climbing, or carries at a conversational pace teach fibers and mitochondria to supply energy efficiently and help the cardiovascular and muscular systems cooperate. A fourth is range: mobility and flexibility used, not merely held. Muscles lengthen more willingly when the nervous system perceives safety; slow, comfortable stretching and controlled movements at the edges of range expand what feels available. A fifth is balance and control: standing on one foot while you cook, reaching outside your base of support, or exploring safely unstable surfaces to keep stabilizers attentive and reflexes sharp. None of these qualities requires a rigid program; they can be folded into daily life as practice.

In practical terms, early strength work can be as simple as standing up from a chair with control, pressing into a wall, hinging at the hips to pick something up with a neutral spine, or rowing your chest toward a countertop. Choose variations where the last few repetitions feel effortful but not panicked; if your breath disappears or your face clenches, lighten the demand or adjust the position. The nervous system learns best when the environment is challenging and clearly safe. As control grows, you can sprinkle in brief, crisp efforts of five to fifteen seconds of a quicker step-up, a short stair burst, a set of lively step taps. Stop before form unravels; rest long enough that the next effort is equally clean. For stamina, string movements together at a pace where conversation is easy and nasal breathing is comfortable. The end feeling you could do a little more; that sense of reserve is not wasted, it is what convinces the body to return tomorrow.

Range work benefits from the same principles. Find the first edge of stretch, breathe, and wait for tone to soften rather than chasing a bigger sensation. Useful places to explore are the fronts of the hips, calves, chest, lats, and wrists regions that adapt quickly to sitting and screen time. Rather than asking cold tissues to yield, earn range with gentle motion first, then spend time near the edge, then come back out and use the new space in a simple task. Balance can be practiced in small moments: one-foot stands while brushing your teeth, slow reaches across the counter, or standing on a folded towel while you fold laundry. These little inputs keep deep stabilizers engaged and reduce fall risk across the lifespan.

A few notes keep expectations realistic and kind. Soreness after unfamiliar effort is common, but it is not required for progress and is not a measure of quality. Chasing soreness tends to produce less consistency, not more adaptation. Progress does not move in a straight line; capacity expands and contracts with sleep, food, stress, illness, and the rest of life. Adequate protein, hydration, micronutrients, and sleep support repair and adaptation, but they cannot substitute for mechanical signals; the tissue must be asked to change. Likewise, more is not always better. Very high volumes or intensities without recovery can increase fatigue and injury risk and, for some, keep stress chemistry elevated. The body learns on the resting days too.

It is also worth naming how "stress" shows up in tissue. When sympathetic arousal is high and persistent, background muscle tone tends to rise. That tone is not imaginary; it can be measured and felt. High tone reduces willingness to lengthen and changes how joints are loaded. Practices from earlier chapters breath with a slightly longer exhale, brief body scans, cues of safety lower the background noise so range and strength work proceed with less friction. Movement can, in turn, soften the nervous system: contracting large muscles and moving rhythmically often improves mood and eases hypervigilance through multiple pathways. None of this turns exercise into a cure-all, but it helps explain why even short bouts often leave you feeling more available to your life.

Because bodies differ, so should progressions. If you live with pain that limits daily function; neurologic, cardiovascular, or metabolic conditions; bone fragility; connective-tissue disorders; a history of falls; or if exercise consistently provokes dizziness, chest discomfort, or disproportionate breathlessness, partner with a qualified clinician. Good guidance does not remove effort; it organizes it. Coaches and teachers can provide technique, structure, and accountability, but no one can do your repetitions for you. Learning from professionals is valuable; applying what you learn in your own body is essential. Health has many determinants: genetics, environment, social context, sleep, nutrition, medical care but when it comes to muscular adaptation, your participation is the irreplaceable ingredient. Connection comes first: if you are not listening to your body's signals, it is easy to lift more, stretch farther, or endure longer while moving farther from what you actually need. Re-establishing that connection through attention, breath, and sustainable effort makes every other minute you spend training more effective.

As you move more often and more skillfully, you may notice changes that are modest at first and meaningful over time: joints feel steadier, steps feel lighter, breath and footfall find a shared rhythm, and daily tasks ask less of you than they once did. Shape and tone often follow function, muscles become more visible when they are used and nourished; posture looks different when stabilizers know their job. None of this requires chasing someone else's ideal or pushing to exhaustion. It asks for participation rather than performance. You are not sculpting a body you dislike; you are reclaiming a body you can inhabit. Every careful repetition says, "This is safe and useful." Every easy stretch says, "You can let me in a little." Every crisp effort says, "We can be quick without panicking." Over time, those messages accumulate. Trust returns not as an idea, but as a felt sense that you and your body are on the same side.

The next step in this healing sequence builds directly on that foundation. Muscles do not act in isolation; they attach to levers and pull on pulleys. They need something to anchor to, to stabilize from, to coordinate around. They need structure. They need alignment. They need the architectural intelligence of the system that holds your frame together, the skeletal system. That is where we will go next.

For now, keep today simple. Let it be one movement at a time, not as a task to check off but as a gesture of remembrance. Let it be a return to rhythm rather than a rigid routine. Let your muscles feel heard, used, not ignored; honored, not judged. The more you move not to fix or impress, but to feel, the more available and alive your body becomes. Aliveness is not a guarantee of any particular outcome, but it is a powerful condition for healing: a body that is used with care remembers how to help.

The Framework of Support

Let's begin with a simple, consequential truth: whatever strength your muscles can generate, however smoothly your organs perform, and however fluid your movement appears, it is difficult to sustain progress without a stable structure beneath it all. Durable restoration depends on a reliable framework, one that bears load, shares load, and transmits forces without unnecessary strain. That framework is the skeletal system. Your skeleton is not merely scaffolding; it is living tissue that adapts throughout life to movement, load, nutrition, hormones, and the rhythms of rest and stress. With every step, lift, and breath, mechanical forces travel through the spine, ribs, pelvis, and limbs. Bones may not "carry your life force," but they do distribute the physical forces of gravity and motion so the rest of you can work with less friction and less waste.

When structure falters, effort leaks into compensation. Misaligned joints change how forces are absorbed; underused regions stiffen while others overwork. Over time, these imbalances, sometimes subtle, can contribute to localized pain, low-grade inflammation, and fatigue, not because you are broken, but because your body must spend extra energy to accomplish ordinary tasks. Even strong muscles will brace and tire if the frame they pull against is unsettled. Just as a house needs sound beams to remain livable, a body needs a dependable framework to make healing plausible and lasting. Restoring the skeleton, then, is not about rigid posing; it is about helping a living architecture regain the adaptability and alignment that let every other system do its work more easily.

The skeletal system is far more than a pile of bones. In the typical adult there are about 206 of them (the number can vary slightly), joined by cartilage, ligaments, synovial capsules, and other connective tissues. Together they protect vital organs, provide levers and anchor points for muscles, store minerals such as calcium and phosphate, and house bone marrow where new blood cells are formed. Articular cartilage at joint surfaces spreads load and reduces friction; because it has no direct blood supply, it relies on movement to draw in nutrients and expel waste via synovial fluid. Ligaments connect bone to bone and guide motion within safe limits. The periosteum is a thin, highly innervated membrane that wraps each bone, carries blood vessels and hosts cells that can form new bone at the surface; its sensitivity is one reason irritated bony regions can feel tender.

Bone is metabolically active tissue engaged in a lifelong conversation between breakdown and rebuilding. Osteoclasts resorb bone; osteoblasts lay down a new matrix; osteocytes the mature bone cells embedded within that matrix sense strain and fluid flow and send signals that influence both processes. This remodeling follows a principle often called Wolff's law: bone adapts to the stresses placed upon it, adding where forces are frequent and removing where they are rare. Mechanical loading tends to suppress sclerostin (an osteocyte-derived inhibitor of bone formation) and support pathways that favor building. Prolonged unloading extended bed rest, very low activity, or microgravity promotes loss. Beyond structure, bone participates in whole-body chemistry. It acts as a mineral reservoir that helps buffer acid–base changes over time. It releases signals such as FGF23, which helps regulate phosphate balance through the kidneys, and osteocalcin, which animal studies suggest influences energy metabolism and perhaps cognition; in humans, the scope of osteocalcin's effects is still being clarified. The point is not that bone controls everything, but that it contributes to more conversations than once imagined.

Because the skeleton interdepends with the nervous, muscular, and circulatory systems, structure rarely changes well in isolation. Bones do not move themselves. Muscles pull on them through tendons; fascia distributes force across chains; autonomic tone influences posture; breathing shapes rib and spinal motion; circulation and interstitial fluids influence how tissues recover after load. That is why the skeletal system appears fifth in this sequence after breath, the nervous system, circulation, and muscles. As breathing steadies and the nervous system spends more time in regulated states, blood distributes resources more effectively, and muscles can lengthen and contract with less guarding. In that context, the skeleton becomes more receptive to the inputs movement and load that tell it how to remodel. Alignment is not imposed from the outside; it emerges as these systems cooperate.

It helps to be precise about what alignment does and does not mean. There is no single perfect posture for everybody all day; humans are built to move through many shapes. Still, the way you typically stack head, ribcage, and pelvis changes how forces travel. A pronounced forward head increases the moment arm on the cervical spine and tends to recruit neck muscles that might otherwise rest. Marked thoracic kyphosis can alter rib mechanics and, in some people, is associated with reduced respiratory volumes. A persistently anterior or posterior pelvic tilt changes lumbar loading and hip mechanics. At the foot, low or high arches can shift how load is shared up the chain. These influences are not destiny. Many people function well with idiosyncrasies but when discomfort or inefficiency accumulates, improving how the frame carries load often helps. Think of alignment not as a static ideal to hold, but as a comfortable default to return to a position from which movement is easy and forces are well distributed.

Restoring the skeletal system does not mean forcing your body into rigid shapes or chasing an ideal silhouette. It begins with awareness and believable inputs that bones and joints can use. Weight-bearing and resistance work provide the primary stimulus for bone strength. Heavy barbells are not mandatory to begin; bodyweight squats and hinges, step-ups, loaded carries, brisk stair climbing, and wall or countertop presses all create mechanical loading that tells bone, “we need capacity here.” Over months and years, consistent, appropriately dosed loading helps maintain or increase bone mineral density, especially at sites that receive the most stress such as hips, spine, and wrists. For people at risk of low bone density or fracture, details of loading progression, balance work to reduce falls, and avoiding end-range spinal flexion or rotation under load for some are worth tailoring with a clinician. Bone adapts slowly; patience is part of the prescription.

Cartilage and joint surfaces thrive on varied, comfortable motion. Because articular cartilage is nourished by the ebb and flow of synovial fluid, intermittent compression walking, gentle cycling, swimming, easy squats and lunges with clean technique acts like a pump that "washes" the joint. Slow circles of ankles, wrists, and shoulders and gentle spinal rotations help maintain glide in smaller ranges. Prolonged immobility deprives cartilage of this flushing and feeding. For joints affected by osteoarthritis, appropriate movement remains beneficial; it does not "wear out" cartilage faster when done judiciously, and it can reduce pain by improving joint nutrition, muscular support, and the nervous system's sense of safety. High-impact activities may be well tolerated by some and not by others; the right mix is whichever keeps you moving consistently without flares.

Ligaments protect joints by limiting excessive motion; they are built for restraint, not stretch. Because they have relatively low blood flow, healing from injury can be slow, and repeated high-velocity, poorly controlled loads can overwhelm them. The most reliable protection for ligaments is strong, well-timed muscular support and sharp proprioception, the sense of joint position and movement. Single-leg stance, controlled direction changes, and balance work on safe, slightly unstable surfaces sharpen this sense. Strength training that emphasizes alignment and tempo teaches muscles to absorb forces before ligaments are asked to. Static stretching has a place for muscle comfort and range, but routinely pushing ligaments toward laxity is not the goal; stability is. Stability does not mean stillness it means readiness.

Posture deserves a compassionate, practical approach. Rather than policing yourself all day, use brief check-ins to notice your "stack." Is your head mostly over your shoulders rather than far in front? Are your lower ribs comfortably settled over the pelvis rather than flared up or collapsed down? Are you gripping the abdomen or glutes to hold yourself, or can stacked bones do more of the work? Small adjustments, paired with strength and range work, allow posture to emerge reflexively instead of as a pose to defend. If you return often to a few cues softening jaw and eyes, lengthening the back of the neck, letting the ribcage sit over the pelvis, feeling weight through the tripod of each foot your nervous system learns them as a default that feels both efficient and safe.

The base under all of this is the foot. Each foot contains 26 bones, numerous joints, and a dense web of intrinsic muscles, tendons, and sensory receptors that constantly update your balance system. Modern life flat floors, stiff soles, and long hours of sitting tends to decondition this foundation. When safe for you, spending some time barefoot on varied but safe textures (grass, sand, a textured mat) can wake up sensory feedback and help intrinsic muscles reclaim their role. Simple drills spreading the toes, "short-foot" work to gently lift the arch, towel scrunches, slow calf raises with deliberate lowering can improve arch support and ankle control. Not everyone should go barefoot; individuals with diabetes, peripheral neuropathy, poor wound healing, or specific orthopedic conditions need tailored advice. The goal is not a particular foot shape; it is a base that senses and shares load well so the knees, hips, and spine can do their jobs with less compensation.

These elements are already woven into the practices you began earlier. Strength work loads bone. Power work teaches the frame to handle impulses and decelerate safely. Endurance work applies repetitive, moderate joint compression that nourishes cartilage. Flexibility and mobility spread load across fuller ranges so no region bears it all. Balance protects ligaments and reduces fall risk across the lifespan. What changes at this stage is intention: you are now seeing how these same movements shape your framework's health, not only muscular tone or capacity. Progress is measured less by holding a posture and more by the ease with which you move into and out of many shapes without strain.

It is also useful to keep claims in proportion. Posture influences load distribution and, in extreme cases, can affect respiratory mechanics; however, digestion, hormones, and other organ functions are shaped by many factors beyond skeletal alignment. Rather than promising specific outcomes, it is more accurate to say that a responsive, well-stacked frame tends to make breathing, moving, and recovering easier and that ease can support many downstream processes. Safety belongs in the picture as well. If you have osteoporosis or a history of fragility fractures; inflammatory or degenerative joint disease with frequent flares; hypermobility syndromes; neurologic conditions; or symptoms such as unexplained pain, weakness, numbness, or changes in bowel or bladder function, partner with a qualified clinician. Structure can be trained at every age, but loads, ranges, and progressions matter.

None of this asks you to hold yourself like a statue. Trees endure not because they are rigid but because they root and sway. Your aim is similar: a frame that feels grounded and can adapt, stacked enough that muscles need not grip all day, supple enough to shift, strong enough to absorb and return force, and sensitive enough to know where you are in space. If all you do today is notice how you are sitting or standing, roll your ankles and wrists in easy circles, stand barefoot for a minute and feel the tripod under each foot, and let your spine lengthen without strain, you will have done something useful. You will have reminded your nervous system that structure is not a pose; it is a conversation your body is willing to have when conditions are kind.

As the skeleton remembers how to hold you not only mechanically but intuitively other pieces begin to organize themselves. Movements that felt heavy become lighter because forces travel through bone instead of being arrested by muscle. Joints that felt stiff begin to glide. Breath can drop lower into the ribs without effort.

Efforts in strength, mobility, or endurance start to "stick" because the foundation underneath them is steady. This is not a guarantee of specific changes by a specific date; it is a description of what becomes more likely when a living framework is respected and trained.

From here the sequence turns toward the system that receives and sorts what you offer it: the digestive system. The timing is intentional. Once breath is steadier, the nervous system is calmer, circulation carries resources, muscles are awake, and the frame is supportive, your body is better prepared to digest not only food, but also experience. Digestion is the practice of breaking things down, absorbing what is useful, and letting go of what is not work that is easier when the body feels supported rather than braced.

For now, pause. Let your feet meet the ground as a choice. Let your spine lengthen without force. Let your bones carry more of your weight so muscles can carry less of your worry. Healing rarely begins in force; it begins in trust. Trust grows from structure. And the structure, far from rigid, is alive and listening.

From Strain to Nourishment

Let's begin with a quiet, practical truth your body has likely been signaling for a long time: digestion is not just a set of chemical reactions, it is a conversation. It is an ongoing dialogue between the world outside and the terrain within; between what you choose to eat and the state you are in when you eat it; between the pace of your days and the sense of safety your nervous system perceives. Signals travel in both directions along nerves, hormones, and immune messengers that link the brain and the gut. That traffic helps your body decide, moment by moment, whether to prioritize taking in and breaking down nutrients or to conserve resources for vigilance and action.

You are not simply "what you eat." You become what you can break down, absorb, and utilize and your capacity to do that is strongly shaped by context. When your body reads the environment as threatening, even subtly, it tends to shift resources away from the digestive tract toward systems that help you cope or defend. Blood flow to the gut may decrease, the secretion of gastric acid and digestive enzymes may be reduced, and the muscular rhythms that move food along can speed up, slow down, or become erratic. None of this is a failure; it is adaptive physiology. In those states, even very nutritious meals can leave you bloated, heavy, or under-fueled not because the food is "wrong," but because your body has temporarily de-prioritized digestion in favor of safety.

That is why this chapter does not offer a new set of rigid food rules. It is not a case for elaborate elimination plans or micromanaging macronutrients. It is an invitation to restore conditions under which digestion naturally works better: steadier breathing, a calmer nervous system, and a pace that allows your gut to do what it already knows how to do. Food matters. So do timing, attention, and the internal climate you bring to your plate. The digestive system is built to respond to those inputs. When you change the inputs with respect rather than force, it often responds with more comfort, better absorption, and a clearer sense of nourishment.

The digestive system itself is more than a tube with enzymes. It is a coordinated network that senses, prepares, transforms, and transports. The process begins before your first bite: the sight, smell, and expectation of food activate the cephalic phase of digestion, largely via the vagus nerve. That parasympathetic ("rest-and-digest") signaling increases salivation and primes the stomach, pancreas, and biliary system to receive and process a meal. Once food enters the mouth, chewing breaks it into smaller pieces while saliva containing amylase and other factors begins carbohydrate digestion and moistens the bolus so it can be safely swallowed. The esophagus then moves what you have swallowed toward the stomach through coordinated waves of smooth muscle contraction called peristalsis. Those waves are effective enough that gravity is not essential for the transit; even so, lying flat after a meal increases the likelihood of reflux for many people, so upright is generally friendlier.

In the stomach, hydrochloric acid unfolds proteins and activates pepsin, an enzyme that starts protein digestion. The stomach is not just a mixing chamber; it senses the macronutrients and acidity of its contents and adjusts both its emptying rate and its hormonal signals accordingly. From there, partially digested contents (chyme) enter the small intestine, where most digestion and absorption occur. The pancreas secretes bicarbonate to neutralize stomach acid and releases digestive enzymes proteases, lipase, and amylase while the liver produces bile (stored and concentrated in the gallbladder) that emulsifies fats so lipases can act more efficiently. The inner surface of the small intestine is lined with villi and microvilli, which massively expand surface area. At the microscopic brush border, additional enzymes complete the breakdown of nutrients so they can cross the epithelial barrier into the bloodstream or lymph. Fat-soluble vitamins hitch a ride with dietary fats and bile; vitamin B_{12}, bound to intrinsic factor from the stomach, is absorbed in the terminal ileum a detail that matters later when we talk about what the microbiome can and cannot supply.

The large intestine, or colon, reabsorbs water and electrolytes, compacts waste, and hosts a dense ecosystem of microbes. That microbiome ferments fibers we cannot digest into short-chain fatty acids that nourish colon cells and influence immune and metabolic signaling. These organisms also synthesize certain vitamins, including forms of vitamin K (menaquinones) and some B-vitamins such as folate and biotin. They may produce vitamin B_{12} as well, but because most B_{12} absorption requires intrinsic factor and occurs upstream in the ileum, microbially produced B_{12} in the colon is generally not a reliable source for humans. The microbiome's influence on mood and stress reactivity via the gut–brain axis is an active area of research; evidence supports bidirectional communication, though specific cause-and-effect pathways vary across individuals and are still being mapped.

Supporting this flow are organs that multitask constantly. The liver manufactures bile, stores glycogen, interconverts nutrients, and enzymatically processes medications and other compounds so they can be excreted; "detoxification" in this scientific sense is not a fad but a normal hepatic function. The gallbladder releases bile in response to cholecystokinin when fat enters the gut. The pancreas delivers digestive enzymes and regulates blood glucose by releasing insulin and glucagon. The gut-associated lymphoid tissue (GALT) rich in immune cells and secretory IgA samples contents and helps maintain a barrier that is permeable enough to absorb nutrients yet selective enough to limit pathogens. The enteric nervous system, a dense web of neurons in the gut wall, governs local motility and secretion and interacts with the central nervous system; it produces large amounts of serotonin, which regulates intestinal motility and platelet function, though peripheral serotonin does not cross the blood-brain barrier to directly set mood.

If digestion plays such a central role in energy and repair, why address it sixth? Because the gut does not operate in isolation. It is the beneficiary of the conditions you built in earlier chapters. Steadier breathing modulates vagal tone and primes the cephalic phase. A more regulated nervous system spends more time in parasympathetic states where digestive secretions and peristalsis are supported. Improved circulation delivers oxygen and nutrients to the intestinal wall and splanchnic organs. Muscular activity and skeletal alignment influence abdominal pressures and motility. When those systems cooperate, the digestive tract is better positioned to do its work without feeling rushed or threatened. Put simply: safety opens the door; digestion walks through it.

Restoring digestion, then, begins not with a shopping list, but with pace and presence. Before you eat, let your nervous system know that a meal is coming and that it is safe to receive it. That can be as simple as pausing for two slow breaths, sitting down, and looking at your food. Devices away. Shoulders are soft. Smell primes salivation and gastric readiness; sight and expectation do, too. These few seconds are not a ritual for its own sake, they are the switch that turns on the "preheat" cycle of digestion.

Once you begin, give your mouth time to do its job. Chewing thoroughly is a mechanical kindness to every organ downstream, and it acts as a signal that coordinates secretions from stomach, pancreas, and small intestine. Eating slowly also gives your gut-brain signaling time to work; stretch and nutrient receptors in the small intestine trigger hormones such as cholecystokinin, GLP-1, and PYY that contribute to satiety and regulate gastric emptying. You do not need to count chews. Choose one meal a day to truly taste, put the utensil down between bites, and let your breath remain smooth. Those choices often reduce post-meal bloating and heaviness simply by aligning your behavior with how your physiology prefers to operate.

What you feed your microbes matters as well. A diverse, plant-forward pattern vegetables, fruits, legumes, whole grains, herbs, nuts, and seeds tends to support a more diverse microbiome, and diversity is associated with resilience. Instead of chasing "superfoods," think "super variety." Add a new plant each week and rotate what you already use. Include a mix of fibers (soluble and insoluble) and, if tolerated, fermented foods such as yogurt, kefir, or sauerkraut to supply live microbes and metabolites. If you have conditions like active inflammatory bowel disease, small-intestinal bacterial overgrowth, or a history of significant food reactions, tailor variety with professional guidance; diversity is still the goal, but the route may be more gradual.

Just as mealtimes matter, so do the times between meals. When you are not eating, the small intestine runs a housekeeping program called the migrating motor complex (MMC) waves of electrical and muscular activity that help sweep residual material downstream. Frequent grazing can blunt these waves. You do not need strict fasting to support them; for many people, leaving three to four hours between meals (and pausing before "boredom snacks") gives the MMC a chance to run. Certain circumstances like diabetes managed with multiple small meals, pregnancy, specific medications may call for different spacing; context wins.

Your digestive system is also tuned to daily rhythms. Gastric emptying, enzyme activity, and glucose tolerance tend to be more favorable earlier in the day, while very late, large meals are more likely to provoke reflux or fragmented sleep. Many people feel better making lunch the main meal, keeping dinner lighter, and finishing food two to three hours before bedtime. Not everyone's work or family life allows this pattern, and not everyone responds the same way; treat this as a lever you can test, not a rule to obey.

Listening to your gut includes more than deciphering food triggers. The enteric nervous system is responsive to emotion and stress; worry, grief, and pressure often show up first as changes in motility, appetite, or sensitivity. Irritable bowel syndrome, for example, involves altered gut–brain signaling as much as altered digestion. That does not mean symptoms are "in your head." It means that tools which shift states of slower breathing before a meal, a brief body scan, a short walk afterward, or practices that reduce overall load can change the experience of eating and the aftermath without changing the ingredients at all. When your digestion is off, asking "what did I eat?" is useful. So is asking "what state was I in?"

Nutrition specifics still matter, of course. Protein supports tissue repair and satiety; carbohydrates especially from whole, fiber-rich sources provide accessible energy and feed microbes; fats aid absorption of fat-soluble vitamins and help with flavor and fullness; fluids support motility and secretion. Spices and herbs can modulate digestion ginger and peppermint may soothe nausea and cramping for some; bitter greens can stimulate salivation and bile flow. If you tolerate coffee, know it can stimulate motility; if reflux is an issue, timing and amount may need attention. Alcohol relaxes the lower esophageal sphincter and can irritate the lining; spacing and moderation matter. None of these are universal prescriptions; they are dials you can adjust while watching how your body responds.

There are also times to partner directly with clinicians. Unintentional weight loss, persistent vomiting, blood in stool, iron-deficiency anemia without explanation, progressive difficulty swallowing, nighttime symptoms that wake you consistently, or a family history of gastrointestinal cancers are reasons to seek evaluation. Celiac disease, inflammatory bowel disease, peptic ulcer disease, gallbladder disorders, pancreatic insufficiency, and pelvic floor dysfunction are examples of conditions where targeted diagnosis and treatment change the plan. "Listening to your body" and "getting the right tests" are not opposites; they are allies.

Across all of this, the theme remains permission, not perfection. You do not need to turn meals into projects or meditation retreats. A few seconds of settling before you eat, a little more attention while you chew, a gentler pace, a curious eye on variety, a pause between meals, and an earlier, lighter dinner when life allows these are small, repeatable signals that tell your body, "You are safe enough to receive." Over time, those signals tend to be reflected in less bloating, steadier energy, clearer hunger and fullness cues, and a gut that feels more like an ally than a puzzle.

Digestion has been working on your behalf since infancy without you needing to manage it. It reliably secretes enzymes, balances acids and bases, coordinates peristalsis, absorbs what you need, and passes along what you do not. What it asks in return is not punishment or control, but conditions: breath that reassures, posture that gives the abdomen space, movement that keeps blood and lymph circulating, and an internal pace that feels more like living than rushing. In that setting, the gut's intelligence is easier to feel. Meals become less about fixing and more about participating in a rhythm your body already understands.

As the earlier systems have steadied breath softening vigilance, the nervous system spending more time in regulated states, circulation delivering resources, muscles engaging with better timing, and the skeletal frame offering quiet support your digestive system can now operate with less interference. The shift you are cultivating is not dramatic; it is rhythmic. It is the difference between forcing and allowing. When your body no longer feels under threat, you do not need to convince your gut to work. It resumes its conversation with the rest of you, and you can hear it.

Place a hand on your abdomen for a moment and breathe. Feel warmth, ordinary, reassuring. That sensation is not a promise of a particular outcome by a particular date; it is a reminder that you can influence the context in which digestion happens. The more trust you cultivate inside your body, the more the system tends to cooperate: meals sit more comfortably, energy rises more predictably, sleep comes more easily. Not because you have conquered your gut, but because you have created space for it to do its job.

From here, the healing sequence turns toward the endocrine system, the network of hormones that coordinates growth, repair, metabolism, and mood. That system listens closely to the state of your gut: how steadily glucose appears in the bloodstream, which microbial products reach the circulation, how much sleep you get after dinner, how your stress chemistry ebbs and flows. As digestion becomes more open and responsive, hormones have a steadier foundation on which to regulate. We will go there next.

For now, keep it simple. Breathe before you eat. Sit if you can. Taste what you are having. Leave a little space between meals. Let your body learn, again, that food is not just fuel; it is a relationship. Safety is the setting in which that relationship nourishes. When you offer that safety consistently, your digestive system is more likely to answer with what it has wanted to offer all along: quiet competence, a sense of ease, and the steady work of turning the outside world into support for a life being lived.

Messages in the Blood

Begin with something quiet enough to escape notice and powerful enough to shape how you feel all day: hormones. They do not announce themselves like a spasm of pain or a pang of hunger. They act as microscopic couriers chemical signals released into the bloodstream that carry instructions from one tissue to another. Because they work in the background, you often notice them only when the orchestration slips out of rhythm: energy that dips without a clear reason, alertness at midnight paired with fog at noon, appetite cues that arrive at odd times, moods that feel less steady than you expect. These experiences are not character flaws; they are information. They are the body's way of saying that its internal communication network, the endocrine system, is adapting to pressure.

Hormones do not respond to force or willpower. They respond to context. They respond to the safety signals you send through breath and pace; to the steadiness of sleep and light exposure; to the timing and composition of meals; to movement that recruits muscle and improves insulin sensitivity; to the availability of micronutrients that serve as building blocks and enzyme cofactors. They also respond to uncertainty, rushed eating, irregular sleep, chronic vigilance, erratic fuel which keeps the network busy compensating rather than settling. This chapter is not about micromanaging hormone levels or chasing hacks. It is about creating the conditions in which regulation becomes easier, not because you command it, but because you stop asking your body to fight itself.

The endocrine system is a dispersed network of glands, brain and body linked by feedback loops. The hypothalamus, in the deep brain, samples the state of the body and the environment and releases signals (such as CRH, TRH, GnRH, and GHRH) that instruct the pituitary, a pea-sized gland just below it. The pituitary, often called "master" not because it controls everything but because it coordinates many downstream players, secretes hormones that influence the thyroid, adrenals, ovaries or testes, and growth and lactation pathways. The thyroid, at the front of the neck, releases primarily thyroxine (T4), which is converted in tissues to the more active triiodothyronine (T3); these hormones help set the pace of many processes we call "metabolism," influence heat production, and affect heart rate and neuromuscular function. Behind the thyroid sit the parathyroid glands, which fine-tune calcium and phosphate balance a crucial task for nerve conduction, muscle contraction, and bone remodeling.

Perched atop the kidneys are the adrenal glands. Their cortex produces steroid hormones such as cortisol and aldosterone; the medulla produces catecholamines such as epinephrine and norepinephrine. Cortisol follows a circadian pattern typically higher in the morning and lower at night supporting wakefulness, fuel availability, and inflammatory tone; catecholamines help you respond to acute demands. These compounds are not "bad"; they become troublesome mainly when the signals that trigger them never relent. The pancreas, a mixed organ with both exocrine and endocrine roles, releases insulin and glucagon from clusters of cells called islets to regulate blood glucose with remarkable precision; it also produces somatostatin and pancreatic polypeptide, which modulate digestive and endocrine balance. The pineal gland synthesizes melatonin in response to signals from the brain's circadian pacemaker (the suprachiasmatic nucleus), increasing after darkness and declining with morning light; melatonin helps time the sleep-wake cycle more than it "sedates" you. The ovaries produce estrogens and progesterone in cyclical patterns; the testes produce testosterone in a more tonic pattern with diurnal variation. These sex steroids influence reproductive function, bone density, body composition, and mood, and they also interact with other endocrine axes. Fat tissue, skeletal muscle, liver, bone, and the gastrointestinal tract produce hormones and cytokines as well—leptin and adiponectin from adipose tissue; myokines from muscle; FGF23 and osteocalcin from bone; incretins such as GLP-1 and GIP from the gut reminding us that "endocrine organs" are not just glands.

None of these signals operate alone. Each is part of a feedback system that compares current conditions with set points and then adjusts. Thyroid hormones feed back to the pituitary and hypothalamus to modulate TSH release; cortisol feeds back along the hypothalamic–

pituitary–adrenal (HPA) axis; sex steroids modulate the hypothalamic–pituitary–gonadal (HPG) axis; insulin responds to nutrients, autonomic tone, and muscle demand. A small shift in one loop can influence many others, one reason endocrine symptoms often feel diffuse. Balance here is less like a thermostat and more like a mobile: touch one piece and the whole structure moves.

This system appears seventh in the sequence for a reason. Hormones are highly responsive, not primary drivers. Shallow, rapid breathing and sustained vigilance tell the hypothalamus that safety is uncertain; the HPA axis obliges with chemistry that favors readiness over rest. Sluggish circulation limits nutrient delivery and signal clearance; even perfectly "normal" hormone levels cannot act well if they do not reach their targets efficiently. Underused skeletal muscle diminishes glucose uptake via GLUT4, nudging the pancreas toward higher insulin output and gradually eroding insulin sensitivity. Bone is not inert scaffolding; it participates in mineral balance and signaling (for example, FGF23 clearly regulates phosphate handling, while osteocalcin's systemic effects in humans remain under active study). Digestion supplies the raw materials: iodine, selenium, iron, tyrosine, zinc, magnesium, B-vitamins, essential fatty acids, and cholesterol without which hormone synthesis and signaling cannot proceed smoothly. When breathing steadily decreases, the nervous system spends more time in regulated states, blood flow improves, muscles resume their role as glucose sinks, structure supports effortless posture, and digestion becomes more receptive, the endocrine system finally receives consistent, non-alarm inputs. Only then does it make sense to ask it to recalibrate.

Supporting endocrine health begins with stabilizing the daily cues hormones use to keep time. Light in the morning, real daylight on the eyes helps anchor the brain's clock and, downstream, the rhythm of cortisol and melatonin. Dimmer, warmer light in the evening reduces the "daytime" signal and allows melatonin to rise. A relatively consistent sleep–wake schedule matters as much as total hours; the body prefers predictability. Finishing meals two to three hours before bedtime lowers the nocturnal metabolic load and reduces reflux risk for many people, which can improve sleep depth and next-day insulin sensitivity. These are gentle adjustments, not rigid rules; the aim is to provide your clocks with clearer input, not to add pressure.

Blood-glucose stability is another powerful lever because so many hormones either respond to glucose directly or are recruited to compensate for swings. Beginning the day with protein and fiber (and including some fat) tends to produce a more gradual rise in glucose than a breakfast built on refined sugars alone. Pairing carbohydrates with protein and fat at any meal slows absorption; spacing meals enough to allow true hunger (without courting extremes) helps reduce the chase for quick fixes; an unhurried walk after eating stimulates muscle uptake of glucose independent of insulin. None of this is about perfection or about a particular body size. It is about quieting the roller coaster so that insulin and counter-regulatory hormones can work without overcorrection.

What you eat supplies the substrates and cofactors endocrine pathways depend on. Proteins provide amino acids for peptide hormones and neurotransmitters; fats provide cholesterol for steroid hormones and help absorb fat-soluble vitamins; carbohydrates fuel the central nervous system and replenish muscle glycogen. Micronutrients matter: iodine and tyrosine for thyroid hormone; selenium for deiodinase enzymes and antioxidant defense; iron for thyroid peroxidase and oxygen transport; zinc and magnesium as enzyme cofactors throughout the endocrine network; vitamin D for calcium balance and, potentially, immuno-endocrine crosstalk. Omega-3 fatty acids influence eicosanoid signaling and membrane fluidity, which can change how receptors behave. Rather than counting grams obsessively, scan meals for representation: some protein, some fiber-rich plants, some healthy fats, some color, and enough total energy. Diversity in plant foods also supports the gut microbiome, which produces metabolites (including short-chain fatty acids and incretins) that can modulate insulin sensitivity and inflammatory tone. If you have conditions such as celiac disease, inflammatory bowel disease, or a history of significant food reactions, personalization with a clinician or dietitian improves both safety and success.

Movement is an endocrine message in motion. Contracting skeletal muscle increases glucose uptake and insulin sensitivity; resistance training supports bone density and can help balance sex steroid effects on tissue; rhythmic aerobic work can reduce sympathetic overdrive and improve sleep; mobility work and breathing practices nudge the autonomic balance away from constant vigilance. “More” is not always better; regular, moderate training usually does more for hormone regulation than sporadic extremes. The simplest pattern, move most days, lift some days, vary the pace and load across the week covers much of what endocrine systems ask of you.

Stress chemistry is designed for short bursts; chronic activation is what frays the network. You cannot remove all stressors, and you do not need to. What helps is adding brief, frequent downshifts: three slow breaths before meals, a pause to feel your feet on the ground before opening an email, a minute of shoulder rolls between calls, five minutes of daylight in the morning, a short walk after dinner, a page of unfiltered journaling when rumination loops. These practices do not fix life. They change the signal your hypothalamus receives often enough that the HPA axis can re-establish its diurnal pattern. Over time, sleep deepens, appetite cues clarify, and the impulse to over-correct with stimulants or sedatives tends to ease.

Rhythm also includes cycles longer than a day. For people who menstruate, estrogen and progesterone rise and fall across a roughly monthly pattern, influencing energy, sleep, pain sensitivity, and mood. Tracking those shifts for a few months, without judgment often reveals windows of creativity, social ease, or steadier strength, as well as windows that suit reflection, gentler training, or more sleep. Aligning expectations with biology can reduce friction and over-reaching. For those in perimenopause and beyond, hormone variability and eventual decline change sleep architecture, thermoregulation, and body composition; strength training, protein sufficiency, light exposure, and consistent sleep become even more important levers. For men, testosterone follows a diurnal curve and can be affected by sleep debt, excess alcohol, severe energy restriction, and inactivity; the same fundamentals sleep, resistance training, adequate protein and total energy support healthier levels.

All of these strategies are about cooperation, not control. They will not override medical conditions that require diagnosis and treatment, and they are not substitutes for care when red flags are present. Seek professional evaluation for symptoms such as unexplained weight loss or gain; persistent fatigue unrelieved by rest; heat or cold intolerance; hair loss or new hair growth patterns; new depression or anxiety with physical changes; irregular, very heavy, or absent menstrual cycles; erectile dysfunction; nipple discharge; significant acne beyond adolescence; darkening of skin folds; tremor; palpitations; severe thirst with frequent urination; or any sudden change that worries you. Conditions such as thyroid disease, type 1 or type 2 diabetes, primary adrenal insufficiency (Addison's), Cushing's syndrome, pituitary disorders, PCOS, and others benefit from timely, evidence-based care. Working with clinicians does not mean abandoning rhythm; it means pairing it with targeted help.

By the time you arrive here, much has already shifted. Breath is steadier. The nervous system spends more time out of alarm. Circulation delivers and clears more effectively. Muscles carry more of the everyday metabolic load. Structure resists gravity with less gripping. Digestion absorbs what you offer it with fewer protests. Within that quieter landscape, hormones often begin to self-organize. Not instantly, and not perfectly, but noticeably: steadier energy, clearer hunger and fullness, sleep that feels more restorative, moods that are less easily tipped. The point is not to promise a particular outcome by a particular date. It is to show how often the "hormone problem" feels less intractable when you stop asking the endocrine system to work against the rest of you.

Think of macronutrients as building materials and micronutrients as the tools and switches that make those materials usable. Think of light, sleep, meals, and movement as the timetable that tells the crew when to show up. Think of brief, frequent downshifts as the permission slip that lets repair happen. When those pieces line up, the endocrine system stops bracing and starts balancing. Messages in the blood become clearer not because you forced them into clarity, but because you turned down the noise that was distorting them.

The next chapter turns to the immune system, the boundary keeper and repair crew that allows you to live in a microbial world without being overwhelmed by it. That system listens closely to endocrine cues and, in turn, shapes endocrine tone; inflammation alters insulin and thyroid signaling, while cortisol and catecholamines influence immune readiness. Now that your internal messages are traveling with less interference, you are ready to explore how protection can feel less like fear and more like wise responsiveness.

For now, pause. Let a slow breath move in and out. Notice one small sign of steadiness: a more predictable appetite, a calmer evening, a morning that begins without a jolt. Balance is rarely a single event. It is what accumulates when your body is given a rhythm it can trust, and the space to reply.

Relearning How to Trust

Your immune system is more than a shield that activates when you catch a cold. It is a sensing and remembering network, your boundary, your early-warning system, and your repair crew, quietly evaluating moment by moment what belongs and what does not. It stores biological memory of past infections, vaccinations, and tissue injuries so it can respond faster next time. It also "listens" to your internal environment about how rested you are, how steadily you breathe, how nourished you feel, how stressed you are and adjusts its tone accordingly. When this system is well-regulated, it responds precisely: strong enough to clear a pathogen, restrained enough to avoid harming you in the process. When its calibration drifts, you may notice a different kind of signal: lingering fatigue after minor illnesses, skin or sinus irritation that flares easily, gut discomfort after ordinary meals, or a sense of being "inflamed" without a clear cause. These are not moral failings or vague complaints; they are messages from a physiologic network asking for steadier conditions.

Although we tend to think about immunity only when symptoms are a loud fever, swelling, or a flare, the immune system is always working in the background. It patrols your tissues, samples information from your skin and mucosal surfaces, clears damaged cells, coordinates wound healing, and stands down when a threat has passed. It is deeply integrated with every system you have explored so far: respiratory rhythm shapes autonomic tone; autonomic tone shapes inflammatory signaling; circulation delivers immune cells and carries away byproducts; muscles and movement propel lymph, the immune system's transport network throughout the body; skeletal alignment affects breathing mechanics and organ space; digestion and the gut microbiome educate immune tolerance; hormones provide timing and context. This is why immune restoration is not merely about "boosting" defenses. An overactive response can be as problematic as an underactive one. What you want is immune clarity and proportion, responses that are accurate, timely, and then resolved.

Biologically, your immune system is an adaptive, distributed network rather than a single organ. It includes white blood cells (leukocytes) that circulate in blood and lymph and reside in tissues; bone marrow where most immune cells originate; the thymus where T cells mature and learn to distinguish self from non-self; the spleen, which filters blood and helps mount responses to blood-borne antigens; hundreds of lymph nodes positioned like relay stations; and extensive immune tissue embedded in barrier sites such as skin, airways, and the gastrointestinal tract. At the front line, physical and chemical barriers are tight junctions between epithelial cells, antimicrobial peptides, mucus, stomach acid all limit entry. If something crosses that line, innate immune cells such as neutrophils, monocytes, macrophages, dendritic cells, and natural killer cells respond rapidly using broad pattern-recognition receptors. If additional specificity is needed, the adaptive arm ramps up: B cells produce antibodies tailored to the invader; T cells coordinate and execute targeted cellular responses. Memory B and T cells persist after the threat is gone, providing faster, more efficient protection upon re-exposure. Throughout this choreography, chemical messengers called cytokines and chemokines carry instructions from cell to cell, amplifying or quieting responses as needed.

A substantial portion of immune activity is organized at mucosal surfaces, particularly in the gut, which represents your largest interface with the outside world. The gastrointestinal tract houses extensive gut-associated lymphoid tissue (GALT), including Peyer's patches and mesenteric lymph nodes, and is coated with secretory IgA antibodies that help bind and neutralize potential threats before they cross the barrier. The gut microbiome, trillions of resident microbes and the metabolites they produce plays a training role here, shaping immune tolerance and helping the system distinguish between what to ignore (most foods, many commensal microbes) and what to address. The exact percentage of immune cells that reside in the gut varies with methods and definitions, but it is accurate to say that a large share of immune surveillance occurs there. The goal is not sterility; it is balance.

Why address the immune system now rather than first? Because immunity is exquisitely responsive to the tone set by the rest of the body. It reflects safety; it does not create it. If breathing is hurried and the nervous system is locked in vigilance, the hypothalamic-pituitary-adrenal axis shifts chemistry toward short-term readiness. In acute situations that is helpful; chronically, it can blur immune signaling, sometimes damping needed responses, sometimes nudging inflammatory pathways to run hotter than they should. If circulation is sluggish, immune cells and molecular messengers reach injured or infected sites less efficiently and resolve more slowly. If you move rarely, lymph flow propelled by skeletal muscle, joint motion, and the diaphragm stagnates, which can delay immune cell trafficking and clearance of interstitial fluid. If digestion is strained, the mucosal barrier and microbiome become less stable, and tolerance can give way to reactivity. If hormonal rhythms are irregular, immune responses may be amplified or muted at unhelpful times. Once you have softened breath, steadied the nervous system, re-established flow, re-engaged muscle and structure, supported digestion, and restored more predictable hormonal cues, the immune network finally receives consistent, non-alarm inputs. That is when calibration becomes easier.

Restoring immune balance rarely requires extremes. What it asks for, again and again, is rhythm. Rhythm in sleep and waking. Rhythm in meals and movement. Rhythm in light exposure and darkness. Rhythm in honest emotional expression so the body is not asked to carry what the mind will not name. These rhythms do not guarantee a particular outcome, and they do not replace medical care when it is needed, but they shift the backdrop against which the immune system interprets everything else. Precision then becomes possible: to respond when required, to stop when the job is done.

Begin with the gut-immune conversation. Calm, regular digestion supports a calmer, more discerning immune tone. Eating without distraction, chewing thoroughly, and allowing reasonable pauses between meals help the gut's migrating motor complex perform its housekeeping waves. A varied, fiber-rich diet consisting of vegetables, fruits, legumes, whole grains as tolerated, nuts, seeds, herbs provides substrates for beneficial microbes that, in turn, produce short-chain fatty acids linked to barrier integrity and regulatory immune cells. You do not need a perfect plate; you need consistent, gentle inputs. Limiting ultra-processed foods high in refined sugars and certain emulsifiers, minimizing alcohol, and using antibiotics only when clinically indicated can support barrier health and microbial diversity. If you live with gastrointestinal conditions or food reactions, personalization with a clinician or dietitian is appropriate; immune clarity improves most when gut care is both steady and tailored.

Protect sleep as a nightly immune recalibration. During consolidated nighttime sleep, especially slow-wave, sleep signals that support immune coordination strengthen, and the body performs cellular "bookkeeping": clearing metabolic byproducts, refining memory B and T cell responses, and quieting excessive inflammatory tone. Aim less for a magic number of hours and more for regularity: a reasonably consistent sleep and wake time; exposure to morning daylight to set your circadian clock; dimmer, warmer light after sunset to allow melatonin to rise; and leaving a two- to three-hour buffer after the last meal to reduce reflux and support deeper sleep. Perfection is not required. Predictability helps.

Invite movement that propels lymph as well as blood. Unlike blood, lymph has no central pump; it moves with you. Walking, gentle cycling, swimming, mindful stretching, resistance work that contracts and relaxes large muscle groups, and unforced diaphragmatic breathing all compress and release tissues in ways that promote lymph flow through nodes where immune cells exchange information. This is not about burning a target number of calories. It is about adding regular pulses of motion so surveillance and resolution are easier to coordinate.

Spend time outdoors when you can. Morning light helps anchor circadian timing, which influences immune rhythms. Sensible exposure to sunlight supports vitamin D synthesis via skin UV-B modulated by latitude, season, time of day, skin pigmentation, age, and sunscreen use; dietary sources and supplementation can be considered with a clinician if levels are low. Being among trees and plants has been associated, in small studies, with lower stress markers and shifts in some immune parameters. Even a few unhurried minutes outside, without a screen can change how your nervous and immune systems perceive the day. If you choose to be barefoot, think of it as sensory and balance training for your feet rather than an electrical intervention; the evidence for “grounding” as an anti-inflammatory mechanism remains preliminary.

Let emotions move. The immune system does not read your thoughts, but it responds to the physiology that persistent suppression can generate: elevated muscle tension, disrupted sleep, and chronically activated stress pathways. Putting feelings into words through a private journal, a conversation, a prayer, a mindful sigh can lower autonomic arousal. So can brief practices that bring attention back into the body: a slow exhale, unclenching the jaw and hands, shaking out the shoulders, allowing tears when they come. None of this suggests that emotions cause or cure immune conditions; rather, it recognizes that honest regulation changes the signals your brainstem and endocrine system send to immunity.

Feed immunity with sufficiency, not fear. Immune cells are built from proteins and lipids; their enzymes require micronutrients to function. Most people do better with a pattern that includes regular protein (eggs, fish, legumes, dairy or alternatives, meats as chosen), fiber and polyphenols from varied plants, and sources of healthy fats (olive oil, nuts, seeds, avocado) that modulate inflammatory mediators. Hydration supports mucus production at barrier surfaces and the movement of lymph and blood. Micronutrients such as zinc, iron, selenium, vitamins A, C, D, E, and several B-vitamins contribute to antibody formation, antioxidant defense, cellular energy, and epithelial integrity. More is not always better; excessive supplementation can cause harm. If you have dietary restrictions, heavy menstrual losses, chronic illness, or signs of deficiency, work with a clinician to test and target, rather than guessing.

As you nurture these rhythms, remember that immune problems are not always rooted in lifestyle. Seek medical care promptly for red flags such as persistent high fever; shortness of breath; chest pain; unexplained weight loss; night sweats; swollen, tender lymph nodes that do not resolve; recurrent or unusual infections; rashes with systemic symptoms; new joint swelling; or any rapid change that concerns you. Autoimmune diseases, primary immunodeficiencies, allergies, and chronic infections require evaluation and evidence-based treatment. Care from professionals and care from daily rhythm are complementary, not competing.

If there is a story the immune system tells, it is this: it learns from experience. It remembers pathogens and vaccines. It also "remembers" patterns encoded through your nervous, endocrine, and digestive systems whether the internal world feels rushed or steady, resourced or depleted, constantly threatened or frequently safe. That is why your work here does not involve overpowering immunity, cleansing it into purity, or demanding perfection. It involves creating steadier conditions so its discernment can return. Safety signals: quiet breath, regular sleep, nourishing food, unforced movement, honest emotion, simple contact with daylight and air are how you say, over and over, "You can respond when needed and rest when it is done."

Take a moment now to feel that message land. Breathe more slowly than usual and notice the softening that follows an extended exhale. Sense your feet supported by the ground and your back supported by your chair. If there is a truth you have been carrying, let yourself acknowledge it without solving it. Let the day pass through rather than gather. You are not asking your immune system to be perfect. You are asking it to be proportionate, responsive, and capable of standing down. That is what trust feels like in biology.

From here, the journey turns to the urinary system, the body's filtration and flow network. Protection is incomplete without release; surveillance is incomplete without clearance. As rhythms settle and trust returns, filtration and excretion become the next quiet way the body lets go of what it no longer needs. For now, allow stillness. Notice one small sign of steadiness: an illness that resolved more smoothly, a patch of skin that calmed, a night of better sleep. These are the kinds of changes that accumulate when the immune system is given a pace it can believe.

Filtering More Than Just Waste

Your urinary system is your body's built-in filtration network, a quiet guardian that works around the clock with remarkable precision. Moment to moment, it keeps the chemistry of your inner world within narrow, life-sustaining ranges: it balances water and salts, clears the everyday byproducts of metabolism, helps regulate blood pressure, and supports acid–base stability. The kidneys alone receive roughly one-fifth of your heart's output and handle well over a thousand liters of blood flow per day; from that stream they generate about 150–180 liters of ultrafiltrate, then carefully reclaim almost all of the water and needed solutes so that only about 1–2 liters leave the body as urine. What you see in the toilet is the final expression of millions of microscopic choices: what to conserve, what to alter, what to release, made by your nephrons without fuss or fanfare. When this system is steady, it is almost silent, and that quiet is a sign of health.

Although it is common to describe the urinary system as a "toxin remover," its day-to-day role is more specific and more comprehensive. It clears urea from protein turnover, creatinine from muscle energy use, and many water-soluble drugs and their metabolites. It fine-tunes electrolytes such as sodium, potassium, calcium, and phosphate; it helps maintain blood pH by excreting hydrogen ions and regenerating bicarbonate; and it participates in hormonal communication. Specialized kidney cells produce erythropoietin to stimulate red blood cell formation when oxygen delivery drops, renin to initiate the renin–angiotensin–aldosterone cascade that helps regulate blood pressure and salt–water balance, and calcitriol, the active form of vitamin D to support calcium absorption and bone health. None of this requires your conscious attention, yet all of it depends on your broader physiology: sleep and light exposure influence fluid hormones like vasopressin; movement and cardiovascular health influence kidney blood flow; nutrition and medications alter what the kidneys must process; stress signals change how the body prioritizes water and salt.

The rest of the urinary tract is equally elegant. Urine formed in the kidneys travels down the ureters muscular tubes whose wave-like contractions, called peristalsis, propel fluid forward and limit backflow. The bladder is a stretchy, muscular reservoir that can usually hold about 400–600 milliliters comfortably; pressure sensors in its wall communicate with the spinal cord and brain, and a coordinated reflex allows the detrusor muscle to contract while the internal and external sphincters, together with the pelvic floor, release. The urethra completes the pathway; its surrounding muscles provide continence under voluntary control. When the whole system is well regulated, voiding feels simple and unremarkable. When it is not, the body is offering useful information about load, timing, tension, or context.

Because this system responds to the whole of you, it often behaves like a mirror. Hydration, meal timing, caffeine or alcohol intake, physical activity, temperature, stress, and sleep can all shift urine volume, color, and frequency. Those shifts are not diagnoses by themselves; they are signals to notice and adjust. In that sense, the urinary system participates in the same theme that has run through every chapter of this sequence: it works best when the rest of you is working with it. Which is why support for this system does not begin with aggressive "detox" efforts or rigid fluid rules. It begins with connection, paying attention to rhythm, easing the body into safety, and letting physiology do what it is built to do.

The urinary system appears ninth in this sequence because it is primarily a system of release, not generation. Letting go of water you no longer need, of solutes your metabolism has finished with requires preparation. When breathing is shallow and stress hormones are persistently high, the body tends to conserve. When blood pressure or blood sugar are poorly regulated, the kidneys focus on damage control rather than refinement. When digestion is inflamed or the microbiome is unsettled, the chemical mix reaching the kidneys changes. As the earlier systems: respiratory, nervous, circulatory, muscular, skeletal, digestive, endocrine, immune find a steadier rhythm, the kidneys and bladder can shift from coping to optimizing. "Detox" in biology is not a one-time purge; it is a continual collaboration among liver, kidneys, lungs, skin, and gut. The kidneys are central to that collaboration, and they do their best work when the rest of the orchestra is in tune.

Restoration here is practical and grounded. It starts with hydration that is adequate, consistent, and matched to context. Fluid needs vary with body size, activity, temperature, altitude, and diet, so a simple way to gauge day-to-day sufficiency is to notice urine color: pale straw to light yellow usually reflects reasonable hydration; darker amber suggests you may need more fluids; and crystal-clear urine all day can indicate overhydration. Spreading fluids across the day generally serves the kidneys better than "catch-up" chugging. Caffeinated drinks contribute to your fluid total but may increase urgency for some; alcohol suppresses vasopressin (antidiuretic hormone) and can promote nighttime urination and dehydration, so timing and moderation matter. More is not always better: very high fluid intakes without electrolytes, especially during prolonged exercise or heat, can dilute sodium levels (hyponatremia). Let thirst, urine color, and common sense guide you rather than chasing a single target number.

Food choices can lighten the kidneys' workload without becoming a restrictive project. Meals rich in minimally processed plants and adequate protein provide what the body needs while avoiding the excess sodium and additives that can strain blood pressure and kidney function over time. Water-rich produce like cucumbers, lettuce, peppers, citrus, and melon supports hydration naturally. Berries, particularly cranberries and blueberries, contain polyphenols that can make it harder for certain E. coli strains to adhere to the bladder wall; in some people, regular unsweetened cranberry products may reduce the risk of recurrent urinary tract infections, though they are not a treatment for an active infection and they do not help everyone. If you are prone to kidney stones, prevention depends on stone type; for common calcium oxalate stones, hydration is the single most important step, and additional strategies often include maintaining normal dietary calcium (which binds oxalate in the gut), moderating very high-oxalate foods rather than eliminating all plant sources, limiting excess sodium and large daily loads of animal protein, and using dietary citrate (from lemon or lime) to inhibit crystallization. Traditional beverages such as barley water or coriander-seed infusions are hydrating and generally safe for healthy kidneys; coconut water provides potassium and can be refreshing, but those with advanced kidney disease or on potassium-sparing medications should use it cautiously. If you have chronic kidney disease, diabetes, high blood pressure, or are on diuretics or NSAIDs, individualized guidancc from your clinician or dietitian is important before making major changes.

Movement matters here too, not because sweating is a primary path for "detox" (the kidneys still do nearly all the clearance of urea and creatinine), but because physical activity improves the conditions that protect kidney function. Contracting and relaxing muscles help venous blood and lymph return to the torso; regular activity supports healthy blood pressure, insulin sensitivity, and body composition; and rhythmic breathing mobilizes the diaphragm, which gently massages abdominal organs and influences pelvic floor coordination. Warm baths or saunas can be restorative for many people and do promote fluid shifts and small excretions of salts and urea through sweat; if you use heat therapies, rehydrate appropriately and speak with your clinician if you have cardiovascular or kidney disease or are pregnant.

Pelvic floor comfort and coordination are often overlooked contributors to urinary ease. The pelvic floor is designed to alternate between support and release; chronic clenching whether from stress, posture, heavy lifting habits, or pain can contribute to urgency, hesitancy, or incomplete emptying. A few slow belly breaths before you void, feeling the pelvic floor descend on the inhale and rebound on the exhale, can reduce unconscious bracing. Gentle hip and inner-thigh mobility work, relaxed supported squats, and comfortable walking patterns help the nervous system associate voiding with safety rather than strain. Some people benefit from strengthening (well-taught Kegel work); others need down-training and coordination more than force. A pelvic-health physical therapist can help you identify which approach fits you best; guessing can lead to doing more of what is not helping.

Daily habits around the bladder itself make a difference. Many of us swing between "holding too long" and "going just in case." Both patterns can keep the bladder and brain slightly out of sync either accustomed to overstretching or primed to expect frequent small voids. Allowing comfortable filling between trips, responding to normal urges without rushing, and not straining to empty help that system recalibrate. If you wake repeatedly at night to urinate, experiment with finishing most of your fluids two to three hours before bedtime, limiting evening alcohol, and making the last meal earlier and lighter. Also consider whether medications (for example, diuretics), untreated sleep apnea, or swelling in the legs during the day could be contributing; these are modifiable with clinical guidance.

Sleep and light timing are part of urinary rhythm. Under typical circumstances, vasopressin rises at night to reduce urine production; irregular sleep schedules, late heavy meals, and alcohol can blunt that signal and increase nocturia. Aiming for consistent sleep and wake times, morning light exposure to anchor circadian rhythms, and a modest gap between your last drink and bedtime support the kidneys' natural overnight pattern. Perfection is unnecessary; predictability helps.

Medications and supplements deserve respectful attention. Non-steroidal anti-inflammatory drugs (such as ibuprofen and naproxen) can reduce kidney blood flow; in the setting of dehydration or pre-existing kidney disease, heavy or prolonged use can be harmful. Some antibiotics, high doses of vitamin C in stone-prone individuals, and certain "detox" products containing strong diuretics or stimulant laxatives can also create unexpected strain. None of this means you must avoid necessary therapies; it means coordination with your clinician, reasonable dosing, and adequate hydration are wise.

All along, it is fine to hold gentle metaphors beside careful physiology. Many traditions associate the lower back and pelvis with themes of safety and release. While those frameworks are not testable in a laboratory, modern physiology does show that chronic stress shifts autonomic tone, modifies fluid hormones, and increases muscle guarding patterns that can echo in urinary symptoms. Warmth across the lower back in the early evening, a few quiet minutes of breathing with your feet on the floor, or writing down a worry you no longer need to carry will not cure an infection or dissolve a stone, but they can help your nervous system soften, and a softer nervous system tends to make urinary rhythms easier, not harder.

It is equally important to know when to seek medical care. Burning with urination that persists, fever or flank pain, visible blood in urine, swelling of the legs or around the eyes, foamy urine that does not resolve, a sudden change in urination not explained by fluids or medications, or new urinary symptoms during pregnancy all warrant prompt evaluation. Chronic kidney disease often begins silently; periodic screening of blood pressure, serum creatinine (to estimate glomerular filtration rate), and a urine albumin-to-creatinine ratio can detect early changes while they are most modifiable.

Through all of this, let the theme stay simple: release follows rhythm. Your kidneys and bladder do not require dramatic interventions; they benefit from steady inputs, clear signals, and a body that is more often in "safe" than in "braced." When you hydrate across the day, choose foods that support blood pressure and glucose, move in ways that keep blood and lymph flowing, allow the pelvic floor to alternate between support and surrender, sleep with some regularity, and use medications thoughtfully, you create conditions in which this system can work with less friction. None of these steps promise specific outcomes, and they do not replace individualized care when you need it. They are, however, the kinds of small, repeatable choices that physiology consistently responds to.

If all you do today is sip water with attention, take a brief walk, and exhale fully, you have already sent a message to your urinary system that recognizes: you are not in immediate danger; it is safe to regulate rather than to react. Repeated over days and weeks, that message becomes a tone the body can trust. Tension softens, urgency often quiets, and "letting go" shifts from something you try to force into something that happens because the conditions allow it. Healing here is not a purge; it is a pace. And when pace returns, flow follows.

The River Beneath Our Skin

You don't feel it, you don't hear it, and you may barely think about it, yet your lymphatic system works steadily in the background collecting excess fluid from the spaces between your cells, carrying immune cells to where they are needed, and returning what it gathers to the bloodstream so other organs can finish the work of processing and elimination. It's less a roaring river than a quiet current, but its constancy underlies how you heal, recover, and maintain resilience. If blood vessels deliver supplies, lymphatic vessels prevent flooding, clear leftovers, and keep each neighborhood habitable. This is the body's softer current subtle, essential, and always in motion when conditions allow.

Unlike the cardiovascular system, which relies on the heart's rhythmic contractions, the lymphatic system has no single central pump. Flow emerges from a collaboration of forces. Small segments of collecting lymphatic vessels called lymphangions rhythmically contract on their own. One-way valves keep fluid moving forward. The squeeze-and-release of muscles during activity propels lymph along its course. With each diaphragmatic breath, pressure changes between the chest and abdomen draw lymph toward the veins at the base of the neck. Nearby arteries add gentle pulsations, and body position as well as gravity influence the route. Hydration matters because lymph, like other body fluids, is mostly water. When you walk, stretch, change posture, and breathe deeply, lymph tends to move more easily. When you sit very still for long periods, brace chronically, wear restrictive clothing, or fall behind on fluids, flow can slow. That slowing does not mean "toxins" suddenly build up dramatically; rather, fluid may linger, immune traffic becomes less efficient, and tissues can feel heavy or puffy, cues that the system benefits from support.

It helps to be precise about what this network does. The lymphatic system is a drainage and defense system. It reclaims proteins and fluid that blood capillaries do not recapture and returns them an estimated two to four liters daily to the bloodstream. After meals, specialized intestinal lymphatic vessels (lacteals) absorb fats and fat-soluble vitamins, forming a milky lymph called chyle that eventually joins the venous blood. Lymph also serves as an immune roadway and meeting ground. As it passes through lymph nodes, cells of the immune system sample what has arrived, trap particles, and coordinate targeted responses. From there, most lymph converges into the thoracic duct, which empties into the left venous angle (where the left internal jugular and subclavian veins meet), while lymph from the right head, neck, chest, and arm enters the right lymphatic duct on the other side. From that point, the liver, kidneys, and gut handle true waste disposal. In a healthy state this all happens quietly; when traffic slows or the load is high, you may notice tenderness near nodes, a sense of limb heaviness, or low-grade fatigue that is hard to name.

The system's architecture explains its reach. Just beneath the skin and around organs, delicate lymphatic capillaries collect fluid. These merge into larger collecting vessels with one-way valves and periodic "checkpoints" called lymph nodes, small bean-shaped organs where macrophages digest debris and B and T lymphocytes multiply and refine their responses. Two primary lymphoid organs educate immune cells: the bone marrow, where blood cells (including B cells) develop, and the thymus behind the sternum, where T cells mature and learn to distinguish self from non-self (the basis of immune tolerance). Secondary lymphoid organs extend surveillance: the spleen filters blood and helps mount responses to blood-borne microbes; tonsils and adenoids (part of Waldeyer's ring) guard the entrances of the mouth and nose; and extensive mucosa-associated lymphoid tissue including the gut-associated lymphoid tissue (GALT) such as Peyer's patches samples the world where it meets the body. Rather than a single pipe, the lymphatic system is a living mesh that interacts with nearly every tissue.

Because it operates quietly, many people only notice this system when it is strained. After illness, injury, heat, hormonal shifts, or long periods of sitting, you might feel puffiness in the face or hands, a drag in the legs, or tenderness along the jawline, neck, or armpits. Those sensations are not diagnoses; they are signals that flow may benefit from support. Some patterns, however, call for prompt medical evaluation: persistent, unexplained one-sided limb swelling; swelling with redness and warmth; fever with markedly tender nodes; swelling with shortness of breath or chest pain; or new arm or chest swelling after breast or lymph-node procedures. Lymphedema, often after surgery or radiation, requires early, skilled care (e.g., complete decongestive therapy) to limit progression. Balanced, evidence-based support means honoring both the system's sensitivity and its limits.

This chapter arrives late in your healing sequence not because the lymphatic system is less important, but because it is downstream responsive to the tone set by other systems. When breath deepens and the nervous system shifts out of chronic vigilance, muscle guarding softens and the diaphragm acts as a reliable pump that favors lymph return. When circulation improves, capillaries deliver oxygen and nutrients more evenly and remove small solutes more effectively, leaving the lymphatics to reclaim larger molecules and proteins with less congestion. When digestion steadies and the gut barrier is better supported, the extensive GALT receives clearer signals and the post-meal flow of chyle follows a more predictable rhythm. When endocrine signals (such as cortisol and thyroid hormones) swing less wildly, background cues that influence vascular tone and immune activity become steadier. When immune responses are closer to balanced neither stuck on "high alert" nor blunted, the nodes process what arrives without being perpetually overwhelmed. And when the urinary system reliably manages water and electrolytes, the overall fluid environment becomes friendlier to lymph flow. As the body becomes safer and more coordinated, the lymphatics do what they do best: complete the job draining, clearing, and preparing the ground for durable recovery.

Supporting this network rarely requires extremes. It rests on repeating small, physical cues that the lymphatics recognize: regular movement, diaphragmatic breathing, sensible hydration, comfortable posture, restorative sleep, and food patterns that reduce chronic, low-grade inflammation. Because lymph lacks a heart, it responds to the "muscle pump." Walking, especially with a natural arm swing, compresses and releases vessels in the feet, calves, thighs, and trunk, nudging lymph toward the large ducts near the collarbones. Breaking up long bouts of sitting with brief strolls, alternating between sitting and standing, and taking stairs when feasible all help. Gentle, rhythmic practices such as tai chi, yoga flows, or swimming pair movement with breath; that combination is particularly helpful for lymph. Soft bouncing on the balls of your feet or, if appropriate for you, a few minutes on a mini-trampoline can stimulate flow through the legs and abdomen. If you have joint, pelvic-floor, ocular (e.g., glaucoma), blood-pressure, or pregnancy-related considerations, choose low-impact versions or alternatives. Simple inversions lying on your back with your lower legs on a cushion, or placing your legs up a wall for several minutes use gravity to assist return from the lower body. In this system, consistency matters more than intensity.

Breathing is the lymphatic system's quiet pump. Each diaphragmatic inhale lowers pressure in the chest and raises it in the abdomen, creating a gradient that draws lymph centrally. Slow nasal breathing that allows the lower ribs and belly to expand, with exhalations a beat longer than inhalations, supports both parasympathetic tone and lymph movement. Even five minutes once or twice daily can help. If visualization assists you, imagine an elastic band around the lower ribs widening on the inhale and softening on the exhale. Over time, this pattern also reduces shoulder and jaw bracing, an indirect assist to flow.

Hydration keeps lymph workable. Like plasma, lymph is mostly water; inadequate intake can make it more viscous and harder to move. There is no single number that suits everyone. Let thirst, activity, climate, and urine color guide you, pale straw to light yellow usually reflects adequate hydration; consistently darker urine suggests you may need more fluids. Spread intake across the day rather than "catching up" at once. Water-rich foods like leafy greens, cucumbers, citrus, melon and broths hydrate tissues effectively. If you exercise for long durations, work in heat, or follow very low-sodium diets, modest electrolytes may help; if you have heart, kidney, or liver disease, follow clinical guidance about fluids and sodium. More is not always better; excessive fluid without electrolytes carries its own risks.

Touch can be supportive, though not all touch is the same. Manual lymphatic drainage (MLD) a specific, very gentle technique used in lymphedema care has evidence for reducing limb volume and symptoms when performed by trained clinicians and combined with compression, exercise, and skin care. Home practices inspired by MLD can be soothing: feather-light strokes toward central “watersheds” (above the collarbones, toward the armpits, toward the groin) may encourage superficial flow. Dry brushing with a soft brush before bathing is popular; it can increase body awareness and feel pleasant, though strong clinical evidence for lymph benefits in otherwise healthy people is limited. Avoid vigorous massage over areas of active infection, recent blood clots, uncontrolled heart failure, or unexplained new swelling; when in doubt, seek professional advice.

Food patterns shape the terrain through which lymph travels. There is no single “lymph diet,” yet a pattern centered on minimally processed plants; adequate, not excessive protein; and fats that emphasize omega-3 sources tends to lower chronic inflammation, easing the daily load that lymph must ferry away from tissues. Aim for meals that leave you comfortable rather than overfull; fiber that supports a diverse gut microbiome (which influences immune tone); and sensible distribution of fat across the day particularly if you live with high triglycerides or reflux so post-meal chyle shifts are gentler. If you have conditions that inflame the gut (for example, celiac disease or inflammatory bowel disease), targeted medical and nutritional care reduces the alarms the GALT must process.

The link between emotion and lymph is indirect but meaningful. Stress does not literally “block” lymph, yet sustained sympathetic arousal increases muscle tension, alters vascular tone, and can heighten inflammatory signaling each of which can complicate flow. Practices that discharge tension: a ten-minute walk, a slow stretch, a written "brain-dump," a deliberate sigh change physiology in measurable ways, and the lymphatic system tends to move more freely in that calmer state. Clothing and posture are small details with outsized effects: tight bands that leave deep marks; chronically slumped positions that compress the abdomen and chest; or always carrying a heavy bag on the same shoulder can create minor bottlenecks. Alternating sides, choosing supportive but not constrictive garments, and giving your ribs and hips space to move with your breath all smooth the route.

Sleep and circadian rhythm matter as well. At night, as sympathetic tone falls and you spend time in deeper sleep stages, immune traffic and tissue repair shift. The brain's own cleaning process (the glymphatic system) is distinct from peripheral lymph, but quality sleep supports both. A consistent sleep–wake schedule, morning light exposure, dimmer evening light, and a gap between your last meal and bedtime create the same background that lymph depends on: predictable rhythm.

If you pause now and let a slow breath rise into your lower ribs, you are already assisting this system. If you stand and sway with loose arms, you are helping again. If you sip water steadily through the day, spend a few minutes in morning light, and let your shoulders drop when they creep upward, each of those choices is an assist. None guarantees a specific outcome, biology rarely offers guarantees but these are the conditions under which lymph flows best. Over days and weeks, you may notice small shifts: morning fullness in your face softening, ankles feeling lighter by evening, fewer tender spots near the jawline or armpits after long hours, a steadier sense of energy. Those changes reflect the same principle that has guided every system so far: the body improves through rhythm more than through force.

What happens beneath the surface will eventually be reflected at the surface. When lymph flows, swelling eases, immune conversations become clearer, and movement feels less burdened. Your work is not to push this river but to make space for what it already knows how to do, breathe in ways that invite motion, move in ways you can repeat, hydrate in ways your body can use, rest in ways that restore tone, and choose food patterns that quiet background noise. In that environment, the river beneath your skin remembers its current not in a rush, but in a rhythm.

Healing from the Outside In

Your skin is not only a barrier; it is a bridge, an active, living interface that constantly exchanges information between your inner world and your surroundings. Through it you sense warmth and cold, texture and pressure, pleasure and pain. It marks where your body ends and the environment begins, yet it never stops communicating across that boundary. What you feel on the surface of sweat, temperature shifts, tightness, oiliness, dryness, breakouts, itch often mirrors processes occurring underneath: the state of your nervous system, your hydration, your nutrition, your hormones, your immune tone, and your daily rhythms. When we pay attention to those messages with curiosity rather than judgment, the surface becomes a teacher rather than a battleground.

The integumentary system includes far more than visible skin. It encompasses the epidermis, dermis, and subcutaneous (hypodermal) tissue; the skin's immune and microbial communities; sweat and sebaceous glands; hair and nails; and the connective-tissue web that integrates them with the body's deeper structures. Just below the surface lies fascia, a continuous network of collagen-rich connective tissue suspended in a hydrated gel-like matrix. Fascia wraps muscles, bones, nerves, and organs; transmits mechanical forces; hosts sensory nerve endings and mechanosensitive cells; and helps tissues glide relative to each other. Hair and nails are keratinized extensions that protect, sense, and assist fine motor tasks. Taken together, these tissues regulate temperature, limit water loss, resist mechanical and chemical injury, participate in immune defense, and contribute to body image and social signaling. Their work is physiological first and aesthetic second.

Because this system sits at the body's edge, it reflects whatever the interior is asking it to manage. Under acute stress, the skin may flush, itch, or feel tight as blood flow and sweat output change. With chronic stress and poor sleep, barrier repair may lag, leading to dryness, sensitivity, or increased breakouts. When nutrition is inconsistent, when gut inflammation is active, or when hormones are fluctuating, the surface may show it through oil balance, hair shedding, brittle nails, or reactive rashes. None of these signals prove a single cause, and they rarely point to a quick fix. They are, however, invitations to look both outward and inward at products and practices, as well as breath, rest, movement, and diet.

A clearer picture emerges when we zoom in. The epidermis, the outermost layer, renews itself continuously. Its stratum corneum, the "brick-and-mortar" barrier of protein-rich corneocytes (the bricks) embedded in a lipid matrix of ceramides, cholesterol, and fatty acids (the mortar) limits water loss and blocks many irritants and microbes. A slightly acidic surface pH (the "acid mantle") supports barrier enzymes and a balanced skin microbiome. Langerhans cells, a type of immune cell within the epidermis, sample antigens and help orchestrate appropriate immune responses. Beneath, the dermis supplies resilience and elasticity via collagen and elastin fibers produced by fibroblasts; it also houses blood and lymph vessels, hair follicles, nerves, and sweat and sebaceous glands. The hypodermis anchors skin to underlying tissues, cushions impacts, and stores energy. Across these layers, richly innervated receptors detect touch, stretch, vibration, itch, pain, and temperature, linking the integumentary system to the nervous system in real time.

The glands are central to skin's function. Eccrine sweat glands, distributed over most of the body, regulate temperature through evaporative cooling. Apocrine glands, concentrated in the axillae and groin, contribute to scent after puberty. Sebaceous glands secrete sebum, a complex blend of lipids that lubricates hair and skin and helps maintain barrier function. "Detoxification" through sweat is often overstated; sweat primarily cools and maintains salt-water balance, with only small amounts of certain substances excreted. The liver, kidneys, lungs, and gut do most of the body's chemical processing and waste elimination. That said, sweating can indirectly support skin clarity (by improving microcirculation and barrier enzyme activity when followed by gentle cleansing) and can be part of a healthy rhythm of movement and thermoregulation.

Hair and nails reflect systemic biology as well as local care. Hair follicles cycle through growth (anagen), regression (catagen), and rest (telogen). Androgens, thyroid hormones, iron status, protein intake, and certain medications influence these phases; so do illness and major stressors, which can shift more follicles into telogen (shedding) several months later. Nails grow slowly from a protected matrix; their strength depends on keratin structure, hydration, and micronutrients such as biotin, iron, and zinc. Changes in hair or nails are common and usually benign, but abrupt or severe shifts merit medical evaluation to rule out endocrine, autoimmune, nutritional, or drug-related causes.

The skin microbiome, billions of bacteria, fungi, and viruses that live on us rather than in us plays a protective role. Commensals such as Staphylococcus epidermidis and Cutibacterium acnes help train the immune system, occupy niches that might otherwise host pathogens, and even produce antimicrobial peptides. Overwashing with harsh surfactants, frequent use of antiseptics without medical indication, or heavy occlusion can disrupt this ecosystem and the acid mantle, increasing irritation or breakouts. Conversely, gentle cleansing, barrier-supportive moisturizers, and reasonable sun and wind protection help the surface community remain balanced.

Why, in a body-wide healing sequence, does the integumentary system come this late? Because the surface is downstream of many upstream signals. When the nervous system runs hot, cortisol rises and barrier repair enzymes slow; itch perception increases; conditions such as atopic dermatitis or psoriasis can flare. When sleep is irregular, growth hormone pulses that support collagen remodeling diminish. When the gut is inflamed or the diet is erratic, micronutrient delivery and immune tone shift. When hormones fluctuate puberty, menstrual cycles, pregnancy, perimenopause, thyroid changes, the balance of sebum production and keratinization adjusts. When circulation and lymph flow are steady, tissues receive oxygen and remove waste more effectively, which shows in fewer feelings of puffiness and a calmer surface. When fascia and posture allow ribcage and diaphragm motion, breathing deepens, sympathetic tone softens, and the face and scalp often feel less tense. Addressing those interior conditions first makes any surface routine more effective and more durable.

Restoring the integumentary system is therefore less about chasing flawless aesthetics and more about re-establishing physiological barrier integrity, sensory ease, immune balance, and mechanical glide. Hydration is a foundation, but it helps to be specific. Internally, drink fluids regularly through the day and eat water-rich foods; let urine color (pale straw to light yellow for most people) and thirst guide you rather than forcing extremes. Externally, barrier repair depends on replenishing both water and lipids. Humectants such as glycerin, hyaluronic acid, and urea attract water to the stratum corneum; emollients such as squalane or triglyceride-rich oils smooth rough edges between corneocytes; and occlusives such as petrolatum or dimethicone reduce water loss. Products labeled "fragrance-free" (not just "unscented") are less likely to irritate sensitive skin, and "chemical-free" is a marketing phrase every moisturizer is made of chemicals, whether derived from plants or synthesized. Choose noncomedogenic oils if you are acne-prone (e.g., sunflower, hemp, or squalane) and patch-test new products before wide use. A simple routine done consistently usually outperforms complex regimens done sporadically.

Fascia responds to hydration, temperature, and gentle mechanical input. It is richly innervated and mechanically continuous, which helps explain why tension in one area can be felt in another. While it is metaphorical, not literal to say fascia "stores" emotions, it is well established that stress alters muscle tone and breathing patterns, and that slow pressure, stretching, and heat can reduce guarding and change pain perception via autonomic and spinal pathways. Practices such as slow yoga, myofascial self-massage with a soft roller or ball, gentle dynamic stretching, and heat packs can improve glide between layers and reduce the sensation of stiffness. The intent is not to "break up" tissue (fascia is robust and not meaningfully remodeled by short bouts of pressure) but to signal safety, restore motion, and allow the tissues' water-rich ground substance to move. Hydrating before and after, and favoring slow, sustained holds over aggressive techniques, often feels more effective and safer especially if you have hypermobility, acute injuries, varicosities, or clotting risks, in which case personalized guidance is prudent.

Remember that skin is a sensory organ. Re-acquainting yourself with its signals calms the nervous system and improves embodiment. Simple practices help: notice the feel of water in the shower; briefly trace your arms and legs with light strokes before bed; choose fabrics that breathe and do not abrade; walk barefoot on safe surfaces to engage densely innervated soles and improve balance; let your jaw and forehead soften when you exhale. These are not cosmetic tricks; they are ways of normalizing input to a system that may have been living in defensive overdrive.

Sweating deserves a clear frame. Its primary job is thermoregulation. You do excrete small amounts of certain compounds in sweat, but the burden of chemical clearance sits with the liver, kidneys, lungs, and gut. That said, regular, moderate activity that raises your temperature brisk walking, cycling, dancing, gentle hiking improves circulation, mood, sleep quality, and skin function. Saunas and steam can be relaxing options for many people; they are not mandatory, and if you are pregnant, have unstable cardiovascular disease, certain skin conditions, or heat intolerance, you should be cautious. After sweating, rinse and rehydrate; leaving sweat and salt to dry on the skin can irritate some people, especially those prone to eczema or folliculitis. Think “sweat to regulate,” not “sweat to purge.”

Touch is a regulator. Safe, welcomed touch can lower cortisol, support parasympathetic tone, and raise oxytocin changes associated with reduced pain perception and improved mood. Self-touch counts: massaging temples and scalp, or placing a warm hand over the chest during slow breathing. Therapeutic touch from massage therapists, physical therapists, or clinicians trained in manual techniques can complement these practices. Consent and comfort always come first;

the benefits of touch arrive when the body feels safe during it.

Nutrition supports the surface from the inside. Adequate protein provides amino acids for keratin and collagen. Essential fatty acids, especially omega-3s, modulate inflammatory pathways. Vitamin C is required for collagen cross-linking; zinc participates in wound healing; biotin and iron deficiency can change hair and nail quality. There is no universal "skin diet," but a pattern of vegetables, fruits, legumes, whole grains, nuts, seeds, and varied protein sources along with limited ultra-processed foods, excess alcohol, and high-glycemic loads aligns with healthier skin in many people. If you live with acne, eczema, psoriasis, or rosacea, trigger patterns may exist, but they vary widely; an elimination-and-reintroduction approach under professional guidance is more reliable than broad, permanent restriction.

Finally, give the system time. Keratinocyte turnover in the epidermis takes roughly four to six weeks; hair cycles span months; nails grow millimeters per month. Improvements tend to be gradual. That pace is not failure, it is biology. When sleep steadies, when stressors are punctuated with recovery, when movement is regular and varied, when meals supply what cells need, the integumentary system often follows with calmer sensations, fewer flares, and a surface that feels more like home. These approaches do not guarantee specific cosmetic outcomes, and medical conditions deserve medical care. They do, however, create the conditions under which your skin, fascia, hair, and nails can do what they are built to do: protect, sense, regulate, and adapt.

In that sense, caring for the outside is a continuation of the work you have been doing inside. Each breath that widens your lower ribs and softens your jaw eases facial tension. Each walk that swings your arms and lifts your sternum moves lymph and blood to the skin. Each consistent bedtime nudges repair. Each meal that supplies proteins, fats, complex carbohydrates, and micronutrients gives keratinocytes and fibroblasts the raw materials they need. Each kind of touch of your own or another's reminds your nervous system that the surface is safe. The integumentary system is not asking for perfection; it is asking for presence, rhythm, and support.

So reconnect with your surface with the same compassion you have offered your breath, your gut, and your nerves. Step barefoot onto a safe patch of ground to remind your feet of their role in balance. Apply a simple, barrier-supportive moisturizer not to hide anything, but to reinforce the brick-and-mortar you live within. Feel the sun in reasonable doses and the shade when you've had enough. Choose clothes that let your ribs expand and your skin breathe. Let your fascia glide, not brace. Let your skin be a messenger rather than a measure of worth.

Your surface does not need to be flawless to be healthy. It needs to be functional, comfortable, and responsive, a boundary that protects without hardening, that senses without overwhelming, that reflects the steadier climate you have cultivated inside. When you meet it with informed care and realistic expectations, it will often meet you back with fewer alarms, more ease, and a quiet sense of belonging in your own skin.

The next chapter turns to the reproductive system, not only as the biology of fertility, but as a source of creativity, intimacy, and energetic continuity. For now, pause. Place a hand on the area that feels most tense: jaw, neck, chest, belly and breathe until the tissues under your hand soften a little. That small change is the integumentary system doing what it does best: translating inner safety into something you can feel on the surface.

The Process of Creation

The reproductive system is often described in narrow, task-focused terms: menstruation and ovulation, sperm and semen, pregnancy and birth, erections and orgasms. Those descriptions are accurate but incomplete. Underneath the obvious biology lives a subtler truth: this system is one of the body's primary engines for growth, bonding, renewal, and meaning. Its chemistry shapes not only fertility and sexual function but also motivation, mood, body composition, bone density, sleep patterns, and how safe or connected you feel in your own skin. People of every age and gender experience its influence, whether or not reproduction is part of their life plans. "Creation," in this context, includes babies and also ideas, relationships, art, and new versions of the self.

When this system is working smoothly, many people sense a grounded vitality: steadier energy, clearer rhythms, and a felt ease with intimacy and expression. When it is strained by illness, trauma, sleep loss, nutrient deficits, medications, grief, or chronic stress, the shifts can be subtle or obvious: a muted libido, changes in cycles, irregular erections, vaginal dryness, mood lability, hot flashes, brain fog, sleep disruption, or just a diffuse sense that the inner pilot light is dimmer. None of that means you are broken. It means physiology is prioritizing protection over expansion, a reversible pattern the body uses to conserve resources until conditions feel safer.

To understand how to support this system, it helps to be specific about its architecture and control loops. In broad strokes, the reproductive system is governed by the hypothalamic–pituitary–gonadal (HPG) axis. The hypothalamus in the brain releases pulses of gonadotropin-releasing hormone (GnRH). Those pulses stimulate the pituitary gland to release luteinizing hormone (LH) and follicle-stimulating hormone (FSH). LH and FSH then act on the gonads, the ovaries or the testes to regulate gamete production and to coordinate the synthesis of sex steroids such as estradiol and progesterone in ovaries and testosterone (and small amounts of estradiol) in testes. Feedback from these hormones, along with inhibins and activins produced within the gonads, tunes the axis moment by moment. Other hormones like prolactin, thyroid hormones, cortisol, insulin, leptin, and melatonin among them modulate this network and help explain why sleep, nutrition, stress, and metabolic health so strongly affect reproductive function.

In females, the ovaries contain follicles that house oocytes (eggs). During a typical menstrual cycle, rising FSH supports development of a dominant follicle; estradiol from that follicle helps build the uterine lining and, once high enough, triggers an LH surge that induces ovulation. The post-ovulatory follicle becomes the corpus luteum, making progesterone to stabilize the endometrium and gently raise body temperature. If pregnancy does not occur, progesterone and estradiol fall, the lining sheds, and a new cycle begins. The average cycle length is often cited as 28 days, but healthy cycles vary; changes in length or flow can arise from stress, illness, travel, medications, thyroid disease, polycystic ovary syndrome, perimenopause, and more. Across the lifespan, the system's baseline shifts from puberty's awakening to the perimenopausal transition and menopause, when ovarian hormone production declines and the pituitary and adrenal contributions take on different roles. These stages are not illnesses; they are physiological transitions that may come with symptoms worth supporting.

In males, the testes produce sperm within seminiferous tubules under FSH influence, while LH stimulates Leydig cells to produce testosterone. Spermatogenesis takes roughly two to three months from start to finish, which is why present-day habits influence future semen parameters. Circulating testosterone shows a daily rhythm generally higher in the morning and lower at night and gradually trends downward with age, though the degree and symptoms vary widely. Factors such as energy availability, sleep quality, alcohol use, certain medications, and metabolic health can nudge this rhythm.

Anatomy gives the hormones a home: fallopian tubes guide the egg, the uterus prepares to host an embryo, the cervix and vagina enable sexual function and birth, and the breasts respond to hormonal shifts throughout life. In males, the epididymis allows sperm to mature; the vas deferens, seminal vesicles, and prostate contribute fluid and nutrients that support sperm delivery; and the penis translates arousal into function through complex vascular and neural coordination. Pelvic floor muscles in all bodies contribute to continence, pleasure, and posture; when over-recruited or under-recruited, they can influence pain and sexual satisfaction. None of these structures acts alone. The reproductive system is integrated with the nervous, endocrine, immune, circulatory, and musculoskeletal systems; changes in one often echo in the others.

Because this axis is exquisitely sensitive to context, the body down-prioritizes reproduction under strain. That is adaptive. The hypothalamus and pituitary "listen" to energy availability and psychosocial stress via hormones such as cortisol, insulin, leptin, and kisspeptin. When sleep is sparse, when caloric intake is chronically low relative to expenditure, or when stressors feel relentless, GnRH pulsatility can slow. In women, that pattern may show up as a longer cycle, no ovulation, or hypothalamic amenorrhea. In men, it may present as lower libido, softer morning erections, or reduced sperm quality. These are common and often reversible signals, not judgments. They are the body's way of asking for safer conditions, more rest, more fuel, fewer alarms before it invests in creation.

This is why the reproductive system arrives at the end of your healing sequence. Breath, sleep, nutrition, circulation, digestion, immune tone, musculoskeletal balance, and skin integrity all set the backdrop against which the HPG axis decides whether to conserve or expand. When the nervous system spends less time in high alert, when blood sugar varies gently rather than spiking and crashing, when the liver and gut process hormones efficiently, when inflammation is lower, and when daily rhythms are predictable, reproductive signals often become steadier on their own. That unfolding is typically gradual, measured in weeks to months because tissue turnover and endocrine recalibration take time. The aim is not to force a particular number on a lab result or a perfect cycle on a calendar; the aim is to restore conditions in which the axis can do what it already knows how to do; adapt.

Supporting the reproductive system, then, is less about hacks and more about rhythm. Begin with cycles daily, monthly, seasonal. Many women find it useful to observe the menstrual cycle as four overlapping phases: a follicular "build" with rising estradiol and often rising energy and sociability; ovulation around mid-cycle, brief and variable; a luteal "settle" with progesterone's calming influence and a common need for earlier bedtimes and steadier meals; and menstruation, a physiological reset where warmth, iron-containing foods, hydration, and gentler movement often feel best. Those associations are tendencies, not rules; what matters is noticing your own pattern without judgment and organizing demands, training intensity, and social load with that pattern in mind when you can. For men, daily testosterone peaks, sleep timing, and training cycles are practical levers. Many men perform better physically and cognitively when sleep is regular, protein is distributed across meals, and high-intensity efforts alternate with easier days. Across genders, creativity and emotion also move in waves; honoring quieter days prevents the kind of chronic overreach that silently taxes the axis.

Shame and fear can also constrict this system. Sexuality and pleasure are not merely recreational; they are biological regulators. Arousal and affectionate touch can reduce perceived stress, increase parasympathetic tone, and release oxytocin and endorphin that are changes associated with lower cortisol and improved mood in many people. That does not mean a particular behavior will "fix" a hormone level, nor does it mean that anyone owes sexual availability to themselves or others. It suggests that reclaiming safe, self-directed pleasure, sensuality in the broad sense: warmth, scent, music, gentle massage, comfortable fabrics, a bath, mindful touch can shift the body from guardedness toward receptivity. For those with a history of trauma, working with a qualified therapist or pelvic health specialist can make this exploration safer and more effective; pacing and consent are central to healing.

Nutrition is another pillar. Sex steroids are synthesized from cholesterol; the body can make cholesterol, but chronic severe fat restriction can be a stress signal and may reduce hormone production over time. Most people do well with a pattern that reliably includes quality proteins (which supply amino acids for enzymes, receptors, and carriers), a spectrum of fats (including mono- and polyunsaturated fats and some saturated fat), fiber-rich carbohydrates, and abundant micronutrients. Iron, zinc, selenium, iodine (via thyroid health), vitamins

A, C, D, E, and the B-complex (including folate and B6), choline, and omega-3 fatty acids all contribute to reproductive physiology in ways ranging from steroidogenesis and endometrial maintenance to sperm membrane integrity and embryo development. Hydration supports cervical mucus, semen volume, and thermoregulation. Supplements can be helpful in selected cases—iron for iron-deficiency anemia, iodine where intake is low but not in excess, folate for those trying to conceive, vitamin D where deficient, or targeted antioxidants for specific male factor issues but these are best individualized with a clinician because "more" is not always better and interactions exist.

Movement should circulate, not deplete. Regular physical activity improves insulin sensitivity, vascular health, mood, and sleep all supportive of reproductive function. The sweet spot differs by person and season. As a general frame: combine low- to moderate-intensity aerobic activity (walking, cycling, swimming), resistance training that addresses major muscle groups, and mobility work that keeps hips and thoracic spine moving. Build in lighter days, particularly in the late luteal phase for menstruating people or during periods of high life stress for anyone. Be alert to the signs of relative energy deficiency, persistent fatigue, declining performance, frequent illness, menstrual disruption, reduced libido, poor sleep and respond by increasing fuel and/or reducing training load rather than pushing harder.

Emotional safety and relationship quality matter, too. The HPG axis is tightly coupled to the stress system (the hypothalamic–pituitary–adrenal axis). Ongoing conflict, loneliness, financial strain, and caregiver burden are not "thought errors"; they are biological stressors that change sleep, appetite, cortisol patterns, and thus reproductive signaling. This does not mean you must eliminate stress to heal, it means building predictable pockets of recovery into real life: protected sleep windows; regular meals eaten away from screens; brief walks outdoors; boundaries that reduce chronic over commitment; conversations that move truth from inside to outside; therapy when helpful; and communities like friends, partners, creative groups where your nervous system can downshift. Intimacy is broader than sex; it is the experience of being seen and safe enough to soften. Bodies often respond to that safety with improved function.

Environmental inputs are also part of the context. Everyday exposures to heat, tobacco smoke, excess alcohol, and some industrial chemicals can influence reproductive parameters. Perfection is neither possible nor required. Practical steps: ventilating when cooking, storing food in glass or stainless steel instead of heating plastic, moderating alcohol, not smoking or vaping, using condoms and choosing lubricants compatible with your goals (fertility-friendly, latex-safe, non-irritating)are reasonable levers. Medication review with a clinician can identify drugs that affect libido, cycles, or sperm and discuss alternatives when appropriate.

None of these approaches guarantees a specific outcome. Fertility and sexual function are multifactorial, and medical evaluation is important when concerning signs persist: pelvic pain, heavy or very infrequent bleeding, severe PMS or PMDD, erectile difficulties, painful sex, hot flashes that disrupt life, infertility after a period of trying, or abrupt changes in hair growth or weight. The point of this chapter is not to replace medical care; it is to place that care inside a wider frame where biology responds to rhythm, nourishment, sleep, movement, touch, honesty, and time.

Viewed that way, restoring the reproductive system is an act of reconnection rather than control. It asks you to notice daily and monthly tides and plan with them rather than against them. It asks you to feed the chemistry of creation with enough calories and color, enough protein and essential fats, enough iron and folate and zinc and magnesium, enough water and light. It asks you to move in ways that help blood reach the pelvis and the brain without burning through the reserves you are trying to build. It asks you to let safe pleasure in, because bodies receiving care send different signals than bodies constantly bracing. And it asks you to allow slowness: hormones shift in arcs, tissues remodel over weeks, and new patterns become stable through repetition, not force.

You have walked through a sequence that began with breath and moved through nerves, blood, muscle, bone, digestion, hormones, immune balance, fluid flow, and skin. By the time you arrive here, much of the groundwork is already laid. You have made room for steadier sleep and gentler mornings, steadier meals and kinder movement, steadier boundaries and truer conversations. In that climate, reproductive signals often grow clearer: cycles that find a pattern; arousal that returns without being chased; erections and lubrication that show up more reliably; hot flashes that soften; PMS that takes up less space; lab values that drift toward balance. Not perfectly, not for everyone, and not all at once but often enough, and gently enough, to feel like a homecoming.

So place a hand over your lower abdomen or pelvis not as a command, but as a listening ear. Breathe into your palm and let the belly expand on the inhale and soften on the exhale. If you menstruate, track three months without judgment and note what supports each phase. If you do not, pick a daily rhythm of rise time, meal times, movement window, wind-down ritual and keep it for two weeks, then refine. Cook a meal with protein, fiber, and healthy fats. Drink water before coffee. Walk after dinner. Choose a touch that feels genuinely welcome. Ask for what you need, or write it down if saying it out loud is too much today. None of these steps promises a specific result. Together, they shift the conditions so your body can move, at its own pace, from defense toward creation.

This is where the "reproductive system" widens beyond anatomy. You are creating cells that repair, words that connect, boundaries that protect, relationships that nourish, and moments of rest that rewire. Biology supports that work; that work supports biology. When you live in rhythm with both, you don't just restore health, you reclaim authorship. And that is the beginning of everything.

When Math Becomes Rhythm

We've completed the healing sequence. We didn't just study the body's twelve major systems; we learned how to restore them patiently, in order, and with the kind of attention that turns effort into enjoyment. At the start of this book, we talked about discipline and consistency as processes we genuinely enjoy and feel deeply connected to, not chores done to earn a later reward. That's the spirit of this sequence: a way of connecting with yourself that gently slows the pace of life until the practice itself becomes your enjoyment. If you truly understand this, you'll see it's not merely a healing sequence, it is a way of living. The deeper you go, the more you realise this is math; that math is rhythm; and rhythm is life.

Now that we've explored how to support each system on its own, we bring the sequence into daily life. You don't need (and shouldn't try) to connect with every system in a single day. Move one by one. Begin with the first system in our sequence, the respiratory system. Practice slow, soft, nasal, diaphragmatic breathing with awareness until it stops feeling like a technique and starts feeling like how you naturally move through the day. When that foundation feels steady, shift your primary focus to the second system, the nervous system.

Try a body scan while lying down, as described earlier: a gentle sweep of attention from head to toe, noticing sensation without judgment and letting the breath set the tempo. This is not “leaving breath behind”, breathing stays with you. You are layering connections, not swapping them.

From there, continue in order: circulatory, muscular, skeletal, digestive, endocrine, immune, urinary, lymphatic, integumentary, and finally the reproductive system, the twelfth. For each one, use the practices from its chapter and fold them into your life only after the previous layer feels integrated. Think of it like learning music: one hand learns the left pattern, then the right; only when both are stable do you bring them together. Integration is the art of adding without dropping.

When you complete a full cycle, return to the beginning. Revisit the respiratory system and raise your level, perhaps longer exhalations, gentle breath holds if suitable for you, or breath awareness during movement then deepen the nervous system practices again, and continue through the same order. Each pass through the sequence takes you a step further, not because you are trying harder, but because your baseline is changing. Early on, the process may feel slow. In practice, progress often accelerates not by skipping steps, but because each small success reduces friction for the next one. Skills compound. The nervous system learns safety; the body learns efficiency. If boredom appears, or the thought “Will I do this my whole life?” show up, pause and read these books again. That thought is usually a sign that the goal has drifted into the future and the rhythm of the present has been forgotten.

This approach is not about borrowing tomorrow's health to buy today's appearance. It is about building a foundation that quietly holds under stress, work, illness, and joy. Health begins to feel less like a separate project and more like the way you move through your life. You stop arguing with your hunger or your fatigue and start learning from them. You stop managing yourself like a problem and begin relating to yourself like a partner. In partnership, change is more likely to last not because you forced it to, but because your body recognised the changes as home.

A central idea in this book is simple and profound: healing is something the body is always attempting to do. Our job is to help it recognise its own capacity and to remove what blocks it. This isn't a promise that we can control every outcome; it's an invitation to work with biology instead of against it. Even when we use medicines, therapies, or surgeries and sometimes we absolutely should support work by engaging processes the body already knows how to run: clotting, tissue repair, immune modulation, neural plasticity, hormonal feedback. The external support matters; the body's response completes the repair.

You can see this wisdom in everyday life if you know where to look. If you touch something hot, you withdraw before you can think, your spinal cord runs the reflex to protect you. Muscles around an injured area tighten to stabilise it, trading a little stiffness for safety. Blood clots to stop bleeding, then remodels to restore flow. When danger is sensed, the sympathetic nervous system raises heart rate, quickens breathing, dilates pupils, and narrows attention so you can act. When the threat passes, the parasympathetic system guides you back toward ease, slower breath, softer muscles, digestion returning online.

Your body manages water the same way it manages danger: with signals. Thirst nudges you to drink before dehydration is severe. Kidneys concentrate urine to conserve water. Skin and mouth feel dry, prompting behaviour that protects your internal balance. The gut also protects you: nausea tells you to stop; vomiting expels what's harmful; and the memory of that experience often prevents you from repeating the mistake. Energy regulation has its own language too. Fatigue invites rest before damage accumulates. Soreness encourages gentler use while tissues repair. Even yawning, whose function isn't completely settled may serve arousal regulation for some people in some contexts; the point is not certainty, but that the body is always biasing you toward balance.

Under the surface, homeostasis hums. Insulin lowers blood glucose after meals; glucagon raises it when glucose is too low. Breathing adjusts minute by minute to match carbon dioxide and oxygen needs, helping hold blood pH in a narrow range where enzymes work best. Temperature is guarded with remarkable precision: in the cold, blood vessels in the skin constrict to conserve heat and tiny muscles at hair follicles contract (goosebumps, a leftover from furrier ancestors); you feel driven to curl up, add layers, or move to warmth. In heat, sweat spreads across the skin so evaporation can cool you, vessels dilate to release warmth, and energy output tends to dip so you don't overheat. The immune system is another orchestra: fever raises temperature a little, sometimes making the environment less hospitable to pathogens; inflammation recruits cells and chemicals that contain damage and begin repair; coughing and sneezing help expel invaders from the airways. These responses can be uncomfortable and occasionally need medical guidance when they overshoot or occur in the wrong context but they are, in intent, protective.

Appetite is regulated by signals too. Hormones such as leptin (primarily from fat tissue) and ghrelin (mainly from the stomach) help coordinate hunger and satiety with energy stores. When sleep is short, stress is high, or ultra-palatable foods are constantly available, these signals can be distorted. For some people, that looks like stronger hunger, weaker fullness cues, or "leptin resistance," where the brain responds less to the "we have enough" signal. None of this is a moral failing. It is a communication problem. The sequence you've practised breathing, nervous system regulation, movement, digestion, and so on helps improve the clarity of these messages. It doesn't guarantee a specific weight or shape; it improves the conditions under which your body can aim for a healthier equilibrium.

This is why our work is less about force and more about signal quality. Slower breathing communicates safety. Body scanning refines interoception ability to sense internal states which helps you distinguish true hunger from stress-driven urges, fatigue from restlessness, pain from fear. Gentle strength and mobility practice tell joints and connective tissue, "You are used; you are needed," and the body responds by adapting. Unrushed meals, fibre, and diverse whole foods support the microbiome and digestive rhythms. Consistent sleep and morning light anchor circadian timing, improving hormone patterns. Social connection, play, and meaning buffer stress chemistry. None of these steps promise perfection; together they tilt the odds toward recovery and resilience.

It's important to say this aloud: sometimes weight gain is protective. The body may respond to chronic stress, sleep loss, certain medications, or past restriction by defending higher energy stores. Sometimes signals are simply confused by the modern environment. The goal of this sequence is not to bully the scale; it is to restore communication so that appetite, mood, energy, and movement begin to harmonise. As that happens, changes in body composition may occur, or they may not, and either way your lived experience of how you feel, function, and recover tends to improve first. That is the right direction of causality.

Health also lives beyond the physical. As you cycle through the systems, something steadier often grows in parallel: mental and social stability. You become a kinder observer of your own life. You catch the early signs of overwhelm and course-correct sooner. You build boundaries that protect your sleep and your values. In the language of this book: you return to rhythm. Physical, mental, and social health begin to support one another like interlocking gears.

So what do you actually do now? Begin with acceptance. Name the reality of where you are without panic, without bargaining. Don't aim at outcomes first; aim at connection. Let the sequence carry you. Slow down enough to notice the signals you've been too busy to hear. Enjoy what you already have, a breath worth meeting, a body worth listening to before chasing what you want next. Trust that attention is not the absence of ambition; it is the quality that makes ambition humane. Focus on the process and let results be the echo.

I'll end with a confession and a gratitude. I'm the one writing this, and still, I struggle to slow my life. Not because I forget, often I know exactly what I'm doing but because circumstances and desire push me toward urgency. While writing this book I wanted to finish quickly. The situation seemed to demand it. I rushed, and the pages lost the quality I hoped for. A close friend asked me to slow down "This is life-changing work; give it time" and I didn't listen. Only when the draft felt wrong in my hands did I remember what I've been teaching. I stopped. I took more time. I began again, gradually, and the work became itself. That is what I want for you: not perfection, not control, but a return to rhythm.

Thank you for reading, for practising, for pausing, for beginning again. I hope this sequence helps you restore your life, not by promising certainty, but by giving you a way to move with your own biology step by step, signal by signal until the math becomes rhythm, and the rhythm becomes the way you live.

Heal not by force,

but in rhythm.

Move not to conquer,

but to listen.

Live not only in survival,

but with room for growth.

Math is a rhythm,

and rhythm is life.